AIDS TO PRACTICAL NURSING

M Stewart

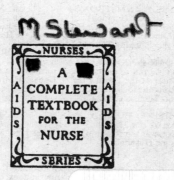

NURSES
A
COMPLETE
TEXTBOOK
FOR THE
NURSE
SERIES

D1181039

THE NURSES' AIDS SERIES

THE GENERAL EDITORS

AIDS TO PRACTICAL NURSING

MARJORIE HOUGHTON
O.B.E., S.R.N., S.C.M., D.N.(London)

Formerly Education Officer, General Nursing Council for England and Wales, and Sister Tutor, University College Hospital, London

with a Foreword by
PROFESSOR M. L. ROSENHEIM
C.B.E., M.A., M.D., F.R.C.P.

Professor of Medicine, University of London Director, Medical Unit, University College Hospital, London

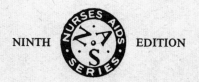

NINTH EDITION

LONDON
BAILLIÈRE, TINDALL AND COX
7 AND 8 HENRIETTA STREET, W.C.2
Reprinted 1963

First Edition, June 1938
Second Edition, January 1940
Third Edition, October 1941
Fourth Edition, June 1942
 Reprinted, April 1943, March 1944,
 December 1944, February 1946,
 May 1946
Fifth Edition, February 1947
Sixth Edition, June 1948
 Reprinted, December 1949
Seventh Edition, January 1952
 Reprinted, December 1952, June 1954
Eighth Edition, January 1956
 Reprinted, January 1957
 Reprinted, April 1958
 Reprinted, January 1959
 Reprinted, June 1959
Ninth Edition, June 1960
 Reprinted, August 1963

PRINTED IN GREAT BRITAIN

THE NURSES' AIDS SERIES

THE Nurses' Aids series is designed to provide a series of text-books in the various fields of knowledge required by the modern nurse. It covers the subjects included in the syllabus of the General parts of the Register and, in addition, includes volumes on certain specialized subjects such as pre- and post-operative nursing, tropical nursing, ear, nose and throat nursing and theatre technique. New volumes are added to the Series from time to time.

Each volume is a complete textbook on its subject (the title "Aids to" indicates that the books are aids to knowledge and not aids to the study of larger books) and is written, except in a few instances, by a Sister Tutor at a prominent hospital. The whole Series aims at providing concisely, clearly and simply just that quantity of information which the nurse needs to possess, gathered together in well-illustrated, easily read and easily carried volumes at a price within the means of any nurse. Judged by the welcome it has received, this aim has been accomplished, and the student nurse has at her disposal a set of convenient, up-to-date, comprehensive textbooks.

THE GENERAL EDITORS

FOREWORD

I HAVE been asked to write a foreword to yet another edition of "Aids to Practical Nursing". Since a ninth edition of this book has now been called for it is clear that it requires no introduction.

Miss Marjorie Houghton is recognised as the leading expert on all problems associated with the training of the student nurse for she was, for many years, Sister Tutor at University College Hospital before becoming Education Officer to the General Nursing Council.

Nursing practice has altered a great deal since the first edition of this book appeared in 1938, not only because of the remarkable changes in medical knowledge but also because of the social changes of our times. This new edition has been extensively revised with the help of Miss Mary Whittow, Ward Sister to one of the Medical Unit wards at University College Hospital, and is completely up-to-date. The methods described are all in general use in the London Teaching Hospitals.

An amazing amount of information on all the practical aspects of nursing has been packed into this small volume, which is a first-class textbook and a most valuable source of reference; I can warmly recommend it to medical practitioners and students as well as to the nursing profession.

M. L. ROSENHEIM

UNIVERSITY COLLEGE HOSPITAL,
  LONDON.
    June 1960

PREFACE

THE Nurses Aids Series came into existence in June 1938 and *Aids to Practical Nursing* was one of the first three volumes in the Series to be published, the other two covering the subjects of Hygiene and Surgical Nursing. The book has now reached its ninth edition and it is a source of pride and gratitude that it has achieved such wide acceptance in nurse training schools throughout the British Commonwealth during the past twenty-two years.

In this edition much new material and some new illustrations have been included. For instance, it seemed desirable to give more space to the increasing number of clinical investigations and tests with which the nurse is concerned and also to include the important subject of water and electrolyte balance. In considering a more logical sequence of chapters the content of certain chapters also came under review, and as a result some procedures which are generally considered to have little value or place in modern practice have now been omitted.

In maintaining a textbook of this nature it is necessary to preserve a balance between the old and the new and some procedures have, on occasion, to be retained alongside newer ones because, though obsolete or obsolescent in the larger hospitals, they are nevertheless still practised in many small hospitals in different parts of the world. Thus, in this edition brief mention has been made of the newer developments in sterilization and the use of disposable apparatus. The introduction of central sterile supply services in some hospitals and the use of high vacuum autoclaves, infra-red hot air ovens, and gamma radiation for the sterilization of materials which are damaged by heat, are likely to provide greater safety in aseptic practice. The delivery of "packaged" sterile supplies to the wards and departments of the hospitals will also relieve the nurse of some routine tasks of a technical nature and should result in more time being available for purely nursing duties.   All these new developments seem certain to become widespread in their use, but since in the majority of hospitals at the present time the sterilization and preparation of most of the requisites for surgical dressings and other aseptic procedures is carried out in the wards, full information regarding the methods still in general use has been included.

I am particularly indebted to Miss M. Whittow, Ward Sister at University College Hospital for valuable assistance and advice in the preparation of this edition and to Miss E. J. Bocock, Principal Tutor at the Royal Free Hospital for reading the manuscript.   I should also like to express my thanks to Mr. Cathrall of Down Bros. and Mayer and Phelps, to Mr. Tullis of Tullis Industries Ltd., the manufacturers of the "Little Plumstead" Hoist, and to the Nuffield Provincial Hospital Trust, for providing some of the illustrations, and to Mr. R. F. West and Mr. D. H. Tindall of Baillière, Tindall & Cox, Ltd., for their ever ready help in the production of this revised edition.

MARJORIE HOUGHTON

LONDON,
   June 1960

CONTENTS

xi

CONTENTS

1

The Historical Background of Nursing

THE history of the nursing profession should interest all those who are about to begin their nursing training. A few of the salient points are briefly outlined in this introduction.

Nursing in Past Ages. Records of the early civilizations show that many of the diseases with which we are familiar are at least as old as history. Ancient India, Egypt, Assyria and Greece gave the physician a place of honour in civil life. Much of the practice of medicine was, however, inextricably mingled with religious practices. In the fourth century B.C. the Greek physician Hippocrates laid the foundation of rational medicine when he stated that disease was due to disordered function of the body, often the result of disobeying the laws of health, and not to the work of evil spirits or the wrath of the gods as was formerly believed. His treatment was based on close clinical observation of symptoms and signs, and his medical notes, clearly but simply written, are still regarded as models.

However, even in Hippocrates' time we find no mention of skilled nursing by specially trained attendants. Treatment was carried out by the physician or his pupil assistants, and the general nursing care of the patient was in the hands of the women of the household or of slaves. Midwives are frequently mentioned in early days, and midwifery was usually an hereditary family profession. The "man midwife" and the obstetric physician were innovations of the seventeenth century.

The Christian Era. The teachings of Christ that service to the very humblest living creature was service to God, and that it was the duty and privilege of the strong to bear the burdens of the weak, inspired the early Christians to seek out those needing help, to go beyond the narrow limits of their own homes ministering to the bodily and spiritual needs of the sick and poor. The Order of Deaconesses was formed and, working with the Deacons under the Bishops, became the first organized visiting service. A group of wealthy and influential Roman matrons, friends and followers of St. Jerome in the fourth century A.D., also included nursing among their Christian duties, although they did not form an order.

In the mediæval period, when the Church was the great intellectual and social force in all the countries of Christendom, the religious orders were responsible for the care of all who needed help, whether from sickness, poverty or old age. It is interesting to note that many of the large monasteries (some housed 3,000 inmates) had houses both for monks and for nuns, and that the supreme control of the dual establishment was often in the hands of a woman, the Abbess. These women were undoubtedly great figures in their day and age. Their knowledge was wide and their administrative abilities of a very high order.

At the time of the Crusades of the twelfth century the military orders were founded. The most powerful and the most famous was the Order of the Knights Hospitallers of St. John of Jerusalem. This order had a "langue" or branch in every country of Christendom. They founded and maintained hospitals first in Jerusalem and later in Rhodes and Malta. The nursing was performed by "serving brothers," but there was a subsidiary women's order whose members nursed in the hospital at Jerusalem, though not in any other hospital of the Order. In the sixteenth century the Order was suppressed in this country, but was re-established in a different form in the nineteenth century. Now everyone is familiar with at least some of its activities, the St. John Ambulance Association and the Voluntary Nursing Corps being the best known.

The Sisters of Charity. In France in the seventeenth century the most important nursing order was that of the Augustinian Sisters. They staffed the largest Paris hospital, the Hôtel-Dieu. These sisters must have been very overworked. The practice, common at that time, of putting as many as six patients in one bed, made their wards very overcrowded, and in addition to nursing they had to do domestic work, including the washing, which they did in the Seine.

Their nursing work was also necessarily limited by the required attention to religious duties, their working day being directed by the priests and not by the physicians. It was not considered suitable that celibate nuns should know much about their patients' bodies or their diseases, so that efficient nursing was hardly possible. The sisters led a life of total self-abnegation and gave loyal and kindly service to the sick, but in those circumstances it was quite impossible that the sick could receive adequate nursing care.

A French priest, Vincent de Paul (afterwards canonized), took an extremely practical interest in the administration of charity both in hospitals and in the homes of the poor, and when visiting the Hôtel-Dieu he was greatly impressed by the need for a more efficient service. With the aid of several influential ladies who had worked with him under the name of "Dames de Charité" in a voluntary visiting service, he took a house in Paris, and there gathered a group of country girls of good character who were to be trained to work in the Hôtel-Dieu with the Augustinian Sisters. His great helper was a Mlle. Le Gras, who became the first Superior of the Sisters of Charity, the nursing community which grew from this small beginning.

St. Vincent instructed the sisters that they were to give implicit obedience to the physicians—this was very revolutionary teaching—and also that they must take no vows nor be tied to a cloistered life, but go wherever they were needed. Indeed, it was not long before the sisters were to be found all over the country, nursing in the homes of the people, in hospitals and in homes for the aged and insane, and from 1654 they rendered service on the battlefield in many campaigns. It is noteworthy that St. Vincent considered that their general as well as their professional education was important, and wished the sisters to have instruction in reading, writing and arithmetic.

The Dark Ages of English Nursing. From the disestablishment of the monastic orders by Henry VIII until the reforms of the nineteenth century, England had no nursing orders comparable with the Augustinian Sisters or the Sisters of Charity. The existing charitable foundations had to staff their institutions with such women as they were able to hire, and the status of nurses was hardly as good as that of a domestic servant in a good-class house. In the private house the patient was nursed by the women of the household or by such "professional nurses" as were available, and there is no doubt that the Dickens' characters Sairey Gamp and Betsey Prig, although caricatures, are representative specimens of that type. The public conscience awakened slowly, stirred by the pioneers and progressive leaders in all branches of science and the professions. The more advanced physicians advocated the training of educated women for real nursing service; the religious bodies, especially the Society of Friends, felt that the appalling social conditions so largely due to ignorance and neglect must be remedied. The latter half of the nineteenth century also saw great advances in medicine, surgery and all scientific knowledge.

Nursing Reforms of the Pre-Nightingale Period. The examples of the communities of the Sisters of Charity in France and the Deaconess Institute at Kaiserswerth near Dusseldorf in Germany inspired the foundation of the many communities in this country in the middle of the nineteenth century. The Kaiserswerth Institute was a new venture that was fast proving itself eminently successful. A German pastor and his wife, Theodore and Frederica Fliedner, had started a small home for discharged women prisoners, and had shortly afterwards added a hospital to their activities. Here they trained a succession of young women of good character and upbringing to be deaconesses. Their duties included nursing in hospital and in the home, home management and the care of young children, and religious visiting. They received practical instruction from the pastor's wife, theoretical instruction in their professional duties from the physicians, and ethical lectures from the pastor. It was an attempt to give an organized training, and though Florence Nightingale, who received practical hospital training at the Institute, clearly saw that the nursing and hygiene could be improved, she was greatly impressed by the moral tone.

Mrs. Elizabeth Fry, of the Society of Friends, knew the Fliedners and their work, and one of her many activities was to found the Protestant Nursing Sisters in 1840. The Park Village Community in north-west London was the first order under the Church of England, but their work was that of visiting rather than nursing. Miss Sellon in Devonport was the head of a band of Sisters of Mercy who gained most of their nursing experience in the all too frequent epidemics. Some of these sisters accompanied Miss Nightingale to the Crimea and were often referred to by her as the "Sellonites."

In 1845 St. John's House was started as a training school for nurses under religious direction, the head of the community being a priest of the Anglican Church. The nurses went to King's College Hospital for practical experience and also received instruction from the doctors at the hospital. Later this order took over the entire nursing in that hospital until the establishment of a lay training school in 1885. The St. John Sisters also nursed in the Metropolitan and Charing Cross Hospitals.

The sisters of another Church community, that of All Saints, nursed in the wards of University College Hospital for more than twenty years.

The Nightingale Era. When Miss Nightingale was asked by the Secretary at War, Sidney Herbert, to take a band of nurses out to the Crimea to give the same care to our soldiers that the Sisters of Charity were already giving to the French, the great opportunity of a life of preparation for such a task had come.

This woman of wide education and high social position had from her youth been imbued with the idea that the care and comfort of the sick and the promotion of health in the family was work for women of character and education. In spite of home opposition she managed to see all that there was to see of training on the Continent. She was, however, to set standards of practical nursing and hospital administration far in advance of any that she found. At the time of the Crimean War Miss Nightingale was in charge of a small hospital for gentlewomen in Chandos Street.

Her first difficulty when she accepted the task of organizing a nursing service for the army in the Crimea was to find a sufficient number of experienced nurses of reliable character, and to refuse the numerous offers from the totally untrained and unfitted. Florence Nightingale saw that this innovation of women in the army hospitals would not meet with favour in many quarters, and she was most anxious not to take the type of woman who would make the work yet more difficult.

When she arrived in Scutari she found a lack of all provision for the care and comfort of the sick and wounded, and an indifference to this dreadful state of affairs that aroused her to a fury of organization and unsparing work. Conditions were as difficult as they could possibly be, red tape obstructed her on all sides, the army doctors resented the presence of women and, sad to record, her nurses did not all prove suitable, some drank, some were unable to stand the dreadful conditions, others found her a hard supervisor and were continually bickering. Certainly Miss Nightingale spared none, herself least of any.

The soldiers looked upon her as an angel, officialdom regarded her in quite another light, but the public made her their national heroine, and when she returned, broken in health, a grateful country presented her with a large sum of money (£9,000 of which had been subscribed by private soldiers). With this money she founded the Nightingale Training School at St. Thomas's Hospital. This was only one of the activities of a woman who was almost a continual invalid for the rest of her life, but it was one to which she gave much personal attention. The pupils in this school were "trained to train," so that they could in their turn fill important nursing posts throughout the country.

In addition to laying the firm foundations of the modern system of nursing training, this one woman was responsible for the complete reorganization of civil and military hospitals, and for many reforms improving the sanitation and hygiene of the army, particularly in India.

Professional Organization. The increasing demand for the "Nightingale Nurses" and the opening up of this new profession to educated women meant, of course, that the profession increased rapidly in numbers, and the question of organization and registration on the lines already instituted for the medical profession soon arose. Miss Nightingale herself was opposed to State registration. She always regarded nursing as a vocation, not a profession, but it is strange that this far-sighted woman could not see the necessity for protecting both the public and the nurses from exploitation by those who were untrained or partly trained.

There is no doubt that the opposition of the most influential person in the nursing world must have been a great factor in delaying this step for so many years.

The first organized body of trained nurses was that formed by Mrs. Bedford Fenwick in 1887, known as the British

Nurses Association. Mrs. Bedford Fenwick, before she married Dr. Bedford Fenwick, was Miss Gordon Manson, Matron of St. Bartholomew's Hospital. The B.N.A. was incorporated by Royal Charter and became the Royal British Nurses' Association. With much opposition from within the profession and from without, efforts were made to get a Nurses' Registration Bill through Parliament, but without success. The first Registration Act was passed in 1901, not in England, but in New Zealand.

In 1894 the Matrons' Council of Great Britain and Ireland was formed. In 1898 the council wholeheartedly accepted Mrs. Bedford Fenwick's proposals for an International Council of Nurses. The object was to admit to membership all national nursing groups which had developed, or were trying to develop, professional self-government and a settled professional status.

The first International Congress met at Buffalo in September, 1901. The General Assembly now meets every four years.

During the long period from 1887 until after the First World War the struggle for registration in England dragged on.

In 1916 the College of Nursing was founded by leaders of the nursing profession and other influential persons impressed with the need for greater professional organization. A draft scheme for the State Registration Act was drawn up. With amendments to this and to the original Bill presented by the Royal British Nurses' Association, a New Bill was sponsored by the Minister of Health, and became in 1919 the Nurses' Registration Act.

The College of Nursing was granted a Royal Charter in 1929; it is now the Royal College of Nursing with headquarters in Cavendish Square, London, and branches throughout England and Wales. A Scottish Board in Edinburgh and a Northern Ireland Committee in Belfast are local headquarters for the Scottish and Northern Ireland Branches. It is the largest organization of Registered Nurses in this country and its activities are many. The professional association department of the College is chiefly concerned with forming and implementing professional policies and giving help where required to the individual nurse. The educational side of the activities of the College covers a wide field in preparing nurses for posts in hospitals and in the fields of public health and occupational health, including preparation for teaching and administration in all these areas.

The State and Nursing. As has already been stated the first Nurses' Registration Act was placed on the Statute Book in 1919. This Act established the General Nursing Council for England and Wales as the statutory body responsible for forming and maintaining the Register of Nurses. Similar Acts established Nursing Councils with the same functions in Scotland and Ireland. The Council also has the duty of laying down conditions for the approval of hospitals as training schools for nurses, inspecting hospitals so approved and conducting examinations for admission to the Register. Separate parts of the Register were set up for general trained nurses and for nurses trained in the care of sick children, fever patients and patients suffering from mental illness and mental deficiency. Originally there was a separate part of the Register for general trained male nurses, but subsequently this part was amalgamated with the part of the Register for general trained female nurses.

No further nursing legislation was enacted until 1943, when under the Nurses Act, 1943, the Council was charged with the duty of forming and maintaining a Roll of Assistant Nurses, inspecting and approving hospitals where such training could be undertaken, and conducting examinations for admission to the Roll. The type of examination which the Council considered appropriate for this type of training is mainly concerned with the candidates' practical nursing ability and is known as the "assessment." Under the 1943 Act the right to use the title of "nurse" was, with a few exceptions approved by the Minister of Health, limited to registered nurses, enrolled assistant nurses* and students or pupil nurses undergoing training for admission to the Register or Roll. This Act also gave the Council the responsibility of registering as registered nurse tutors those nurses who are qualified in teaching in schools of nursing. In 1949 further nursing legislation was enacted, and this Act was designed primarily to "improve the training of nurses for the sick." The main provisions of the Act as it affects nursing training were to give further powers to the General Nursing

*Under the Nurses (Amendment) Act, 1961, the title was changed to "Enrolled Nurse", omitting the word "Assistant."

Council; to enlarge the representation on the Council, and to set up, in each of the Regional Hospital Areas, Area Nurse Training Committees which are concerned with regional matters relating to the training of nurses. One provision at least partially implemented a recommendation of both the Athlone and the Horder Committees, namely, the separation of finance required for the education and training of nurses from the expenditure required for the maintenance of the hospital services. In 1957 a further Act consolidated the previous three Nursing Acts of 1919, 1943 and 1949.

It should be noted that the duties and responsibilities of the Council are clearly defined and limited by Act of Parliament and by Statutory Rules approved by the Minister of Health.

In 1937 an Inter-Departmental Committee on Nursing Services was set up by the Minister of Health and the President of the Board (now the Ministry) of Education. An interim report was published in 1939 and contained many valuable recommendations for the improvement of recruitment to the profession, and of conditions within the profession, such as the setting up of a Recruitment Centre and the establishment of national scales of salaries for nurses. The outbreak of the Second World War interrupted the work of this committee, but in 1941 the Minister of Health set up a committee under the chairmanship of Lord Rushcliffe to draw up agreed scales of salaries and emoluments for State Registered Nurses employed in England and Wales, and for student nurses in hospitals approved as training schools by the General Nursing Council for England and Wales. The terms of reference were later widened to include nurses in the Public Health field, nurses trained in, or in training for, tuberculosis nursing, assistant nurses and nurses employed in mental hospitals. A similar committee was appointed in Scotland. The recommendations of these committees were accepted by the Government and a part of the extra cost involved was borne by the Treasury. The principle of nationally negotiated salaries and conditions of service for nurses in the hospitals and health services is now carried on by the Functional Whitley Council for Nurses and Midwives composed jointly of a Management Side and a Staff Side.

The implementation of the National Health Service Act on July 5th, 1948, brought all hospitals, with a few exceptions, under State ownership. Under this Act every man, woman

and child in the country is entitled to medical attention and
hospital treatment as and when required.   The great majority
of the population between the ages of 15 and 65 years are
either self-employed or working for an employer and therefore pay weekly social insurance contributions.   Although
only a part of the total sum collected from this source is
allocated to the Health Service, medical and nursing treatment is available without further cost to the individual.   The
full cost of the National Health Service represents a very
considerable proportion of the total national income, but no
one would argue against its importance for the nation and the
individual.   We have accepted this financial burden as right
and necessary both as a means of alleviating suffering and
promoting a standard of health which is vital for the future
well-being of the nation.   It is, however, the duty of all who
participate in this work not only to endeavour to foster and
maintain high standards of service but also to accept
responsibility for ensuring that the nation's money is
expended to the best advantage.

Mental Health.   The treatment and care of persons suffering from mental illness or mental deficiency was, even at the
beginning of the century, largely limited to custodial care
which had as its object preventing the patient from harming
himself or other people.   The admission of patients and the
administration of mental institutions were largely dictated by
Acts of Parliament, the Lunacy and Mental Treatment Acts
of 1890 to 1930 and the Mental Deficiency Acts of 1913 to
1938.   Towards the end of the last century the Royal
Medico-Psychological Association, a professional association
of doctors primarily concerned with and interested in the
treatment of mental illness and mental deficiency, initiated a
course of training and an examination for men and women
working in mental and mental deficiency hospitals and at
that time referred to as "attendants."   This step marks the
beginning of true professional nursing in these fields.   Since
then great advances have been made not only in the medical
treatment but also in the nursing care of the mentally
disordered.   As interest in and knowledge of mental illness
increased so the old conditions in the asylums, with their
padded cells, strait-jackets and locked doors, have given way
to the development of the modern conception of the mental
hospital as a "therapeutic community."   The psychological,

physical and social methods used in the treatment of mental patients now makes this a field of service for the nurse where kindness, intelligent understanding sympathy and an ability to form good personal relationships are of outstanding importance.

The Mental Health Act, 1959, envisages considerable changes and progress in the treatment of the mentally disordered in the community and in hospital.

Although special parts of the Register for nurses trained in mental and mental deficiency nursing were set up when the Register of Nurses was established, the Royal Medico-Psychological Association continued to be a recognized body concerned with the training and examination of nurses in this field. However, in 1947 the Association agreed that they would cease to carry out this function and that the General Nursing Council should be the sole body concerned with the training and examinations for the certificates of mental and mental deficiency nursing. When this change took place it was also agreed that nurses who had trained under the auspices of the Association and held the Association's certificate would be entitled to apply to be registered with the General Nursing Council without undergoing further training or examinations.

2

The Hospital and the Community: The Hospital and the Patient: Nursing Ethics: Hospital Etiquette

The Hospital and the Community

IN the first chapter we tried to indicate in outline how the nursing profession has grown through the ages, sometimes making great strides forward and at other times apparently lost in an age of general indifference to the welfare of the "common man." Just as the progress of nursing has reflected the social outlook of a particular age or century, so also have the hospitals and the health and welfare services.

Student nurses at the time of entry to the training school have to adjust themselves to new surroundings and may be somewhat bewildered by the many aspects of hospital life. The student may also have preconceived ideas about the hospital and about nursing, which bear little resemblance to reality. It may be worth while, therefore to consider very briefly the function of the hospital in the community at the present time.

First we think of the day-to-day function of caring for the sick who lie in the beds in the wards or enter the casualty or out-patient departments. The hospital has to carry on its work throughout the day and night. There can be no moment in the twenty-four hours when the sick are not in need of medical attention and nursing care. This affects not only the medical and nursing staffs but also the ancillary staff and lay workers; porters, orderlies and domestic workers must be available for a twenty-four hour service, and other departments ancillary to medicine, such as dispensaries, laboratories, X-ray and physiotherapy departments, though not always providing a twenty-four hour service, have to cover a long span of hours and often to work at week-ends. These examples will serve to show that the organization of a hospital is of necessity complex and makes demands upon its personnel that are not equalled in many other spheres.

We must also consider the educational function of the hospital. In many of our larger hospitals, in addition to the training of nurses, the professional education of doctors, radiographers, physiotherapists, midwives and social workers is carried out. Many hospitals take part in the post-graduate training of medical specialists, although not forming part of an undergraduate medical school. Whatever the part played by the individual hospital in professional education we should not forget the role of the hospitals as health education centres. The aim of treatment is not only to cure or arrest disease but to restore the patient as far as possible to full activity. The co-operation of the patient is needed and he must be informed and instructed so that he can play his part in his own recovery and subsequent welfare.

A third function of the hospital is as an institution for clinical research. Research begins in the laboratory, but discoveries have to be put to the test if they are to have any practical use. In the last century Joseph Lister had theories about safe surgery which would abolish "hospital gangrene" and septicæmia, from which so many patients died in hospital in spite of surgical skill. If, in the face of much opposition and scepticism, he had not had the courage to put his theories into practice "antiseptic surgery" which opened the door to the great surgical advances of the twentieth century, would have been delayed for many years. From the days of Lister's triumphant vindication of his methods, research workers and clinical practitioners have striven to improve on this first great advance in the practice of safe surgery, until in this decade we have seen the discovery of chemical substances which can control sepsis to a degree undreamt of at the beginning of the century. Present-day methods of surgery are a great advance upon the cruder methods of antiseptic surgery, but Lister's work was the starting point. There are many examples which could be quoted to show that the close collaboration between the laboratory worker and the clinical worker in mitigating the sufferings of mankind is truly a part of the hospital service. The nurse is a part of the clinical research team, a team in which habits of accurate recording, observation and meticulous attention to detail are the first essentials.

The Hospital and the Individual Patient

Florence Nightingale once said that the hospital should "do the sick no harm." This somewhat sobering statement is well worth careful consideration. Constant vigilance is needed in all medical and nursing procedures in order that these may be carried out with the highest possible degree of competence. A hospital also needs to lay down and to demand strict observance of regulations designed to protect the patient, as for example in the storage, checking and administration of dangerous drugs, and in the measures necessary to prevent cross-infection in hospital wards. There are also less tangible dangers from which we have to guard the patient to the very utmost of our ability. The separation of a young child from his mother when admitted to a hospital ward, at a time when security and a link with familiar surroundings are most needed, is now recognized as a source of harm to the child which may have lasting effects. It has become the practice of most hospitals to allow the mother to be with her sick child as much as possible and in some instances to help with the care of the child.

Older patients too may have many difficulties in adjusting themselves to the strange and even alarming hospital surroundings and the ward routine. They may be apprehensive about their illness and even more about their dependence on others, particularly the nursing staff, which has been forced upon them by a physical condition. In acute illness most patients will passively accept the necessary return to a childish routine in such matters as being fed, washed and attended to in various ways, but some may resent such attentions very strongly and it is most important to realize this and to explain to the patient not only what the nurse is about to do but the reasons why this particular treatment or attention is necessary. If in addition we consider the burden of anxiety about his family and his work that the patient may be carrying, it is readily realized that mental rest and comfort are at least as important to his recovery as the relief of physical discomfort. Reassurance, explanation and information are all needed, and it is the nursing staff who will supply these to a large extent, remembering that medical details concerning the patient's treatment and the course of his disease will be supplied by the doctor. Confidence in all who look after him during his stay in hospital is a great help towards recovery, and since the nurse is the person who has the most intimate and prolonged contact with the patient the effects of her attitude, her words and her actions have great weight.

Many hospitals issue a booklet of useful information to each patient on his admission, telling him about the hospital and the people who are there to help him and including such items as the times of collection and delivery of letters, the visits of the hospital librarian and the hours of opening of the hospital "shop."

If we remember that the patient is one of a family group from which he has been separated in circumstances of considerable anxiety and stress, we shall realize that his illness and consequent admission to hospital have had distressing effects on normal family life. It is sometimes said that the patient is co-operative, but that the relatives are "difficult." This attitude of the patient's relatives is very understandable; even if the illness is a comparatively trivial one it has disrupted the family and introduced an element of anxiety which is concerned not only with the illness but also with the absence of the father or the mother from the family group. When the patient is visited in the strange surroundings of a hospital ward his relatives may doubt whether these strangers into whose care they have entrusted their invalid are really friendly and sympathetic in their treatment of one sick person amongst so many. To watch an experienced and sympathetic ward sister set about the task of allaying the fears of anxious relatives and establishing their confidence in the hospital and the staff is a most valuable lesson in good human relationships.

Nursing Ethics

Ethics means a code of moral behaviour, and under the term "Ethics of Nursing" are included the moral qualities and rules of conduct relating especially to nursing. The word "nursing" means nourishing; therefore it has come to mean tending and helping all who need it, especially the sick. The object in training nurses is to provide an adequate service to tend the sick and to help in the preservation and promotion of the health of the community in general.

Those who enter this profession must have a real desire to do the work and be physically and mentally healthy.

Many qualities of character and mind must be developed or acquired during the period of training. Kindliness, sympathy and a cheerful pleasant manner are essential for the successful management of the sick person and his anxious relations, although the nurse must learn to be firm when necessary for the patient's good.

She is expected to show loyalty and obedience to all those in authority, recognizing that they have had the experience fitting them for such positions. She must show loyalty to her patients by giving ungrudging service and by respecting their confidences and their private affairs, reporting to the sister all matters that might influence the patient's condition, but not discussing these things with others outside the ward.

Trustworthiness and reliability in all matters, however small, should be her aim. These qualities are essential if the nurse is to develop a sense of responsibility both as an individual and as a member of a team.

She should be ready to accept guidance, and when necessary correction, in the right spirit, using all opportunities to increase her knowledge. No progress is possible without perseverance and self-control. She should cultivate the true professional spirit that shows itself in friendliness without familiarity, and in a readiness to minister to all who need her care without regard to social distinctions, race or creed.

These are the foundations, yet more abilities and qualities must be developed in the course of training and experience; keen alert powers of observation, the exercise of judgment, discrimination and foresight, swift action in emergencies, accuracy in all statements and records, ability to organize and to work with other people so that all matters affecting the welfare of the sick run smoothly.

Professional Etiquette

Etiquette is the code of manners or the ceremonial observed in certain circumstances.

It is essential to have certain rules of behaviour laid down in a service where discipline and orderliness are necessary for the welfare and safety of the patients for whom the hospital exists, and where the prompt carrying out of orders by the right person is of prime importance.

The newcomer to hospital life may find such ceremonial

strange at first, but she will soon realize that after all it is very little more than the application of ordinary good manners to special circumstances. Physicians and surgeons of the visiting staff are addressed as Doctor, Mr. (or Miss) as appropriate, the resident or "house" staff usually as Mr. or Miss ——; the nursing staff should be given their proper title of Matron, Sister or Nurse. Care should be taken to address patients by their correct names.

Courtesy to visitors is a point of good manners that sometimes gets neglected in the rush of a busy ward, and such a lapse is likely to make a very bad impression. Visitors should always be attended to promptly and pleasantly; if they have to be kept waiting, seats should be provided. Patients' friends should not be admitted without permission unless it is the regular visiting hour.

If a member of the medical staff, the matron or a minister of religion comes to the ward, the sister or senior nurse on duty should be informed immediately.

It is not good manners, therefore not etiquette, to remain seated when spoken to by one of higher rank, nor to lean against the furniture when so addressed. It is good manners and saves confusion and noise if senior people are allowed to pass first; it is courteous to open doors for them. All these small acts of deference should be done unobtrusively and as a matter of course.

The hospital authorities may decide that certain rules and regulations must be kept in the wards and in the Nurses' Home. A little thought should convince the student nurse that these are designed either for the protection of the patients or the welfare of residents. Rules may at times appear inconsistent with personal convenience, but if we are to establish satisfactory relations in the community in which we live, whether inside a hospital or outside, we have to learn to consider the convenience of others.

3

Domestic Ward Management

THE student nurse in the preliminary training course is taught the methods and practice of domestic cleaning. In the hospital wards the routine daily cleaning is carried out by domestic workers, but the nurse must be familiar with proper methods of cleaning so that she can efficiently supervise the domestic staff. While it is accepted that the nurse should be freed from extraneous tasks which prevent her from giving her full time to the nursing care of her patients, it remains her responsibility to see that the patients' environment is clean, orderly and cheerful.

Rules to be observed in Cleaning

(1) All articles required should be collected before beginning.

(2) Clean dusters, rubbers and brushes, and clean water must be used.

(3) Sweeping should be done before dusting, with the exception of the "high dusting" of walls, ledges, blinds, etc.

(4) In order to avoid scattering the dust a damp duster should be used for hospital furniture. Polished surfaces will not be harmed by this treatment if a soft dry cloth is used afterwards to restore the polish.

(5) Dusting should be done with firm, even strokes, starting at the top.

(6) Furniture polish, preferably liquid, should be used sparingly once a week on polished furniture and surfaces.

(7) Paint work should be washed with water containing a small quantity of detergent or soap powder. Cleaning powders should only be used when necessary to remove marks, as they will always remove some of the paint.

(8) Method and thoroughness must be practised, otherwise corners and ledges may be omitted, and time and energy are wasted in covering the same ground again.

(9) All cleaning should be done as quietly and with as little disturbance of the patients as possible. Furniture should be returned to its place as it is dusted, so that the ward presents a tidy appearance.

(10) All rubbish must be collected from tables and patients' lockers when they are dusted in the early morning and during the day.

(11) The insides of lockers must be periodically inspected, tidied and scrubbed. The nurses are responsible for seeing that patients do not keep forbidden articles in their lockers, but no article belonging to a patient may be thrown away without permission.

(12) Care and economy must be practised in the use of cleaning materials. In addition to being wasteful, the too free use of soap, soda and cleaning powders is harmful to painted woodwork, polished surfaces and porcelain glaze. Detergent powders and solutions are also harmful to the skin if used in too strong a concentration.

Walls

Ward and annexe walls must be washable. Glossy paint is most often used for the wards and paint or tiles for the annexes. A wall brush may be used or a cloth tied to a light broom for the routine dusting. Periodic wall washing is usually done by male cleaners, and the frequency with which this is done will depend on the type of material and the use of the room; for example, the walls of an operating theatre are usually washed daily.

Floors

Suitable types of flooring for wards and annexes are terrazzo, hardwood, linoleum, rubber and quarry tiles. "Softwood" floors, being porous, should have a covering of non-porous material.

Tiled or terrazzo floors are scrubbed with yellow soap and water. Rubber and linoleum can be washed with soap and water but should be well dried afterwards. Wood block floors are usually polished but need occasional washing. Any water spilt on a polished floor should be wiped up at once, not only will the polished surface be spoilt but the floor is made dangerously slippery.

Efforts to reduce the number of bacteria in the air of the

ward include the treatment of certain types of floors with spindle oil. Oiled floors minimize the amount of dust carried into the air by sweeping and traffic through the ward. Spindle oil is a crude petroleum oil which can be applied to linoleum or wooden floors but should not be used for rubber. It is not suitable for cement floors as it sinks into the floor too rapidly to be effective in holding the dust. The floor should be scrubbed before the oiling. The spindle oil should be thinly applied using a floor mop. Two subsequent applications should be made at intervals of two and then fifteen weeks. After this treatment re-oiling should be carried out at seven-week intervals. The staff and ambulant patients should be warned that floors treated with spindle oil are slippery for a few hours after the application.

Unless the floor cleaning is carried out with a vacuum cleaner moist sawdust or tea-leaves should be scattered on the floor before sweeping to prevent the dust from rising.

Vacuum cleaners and electric polishers are in common use in hospitals. The nurse should be familiar with the operation of the particular type used, so that she is able to see that domestic staff use the apparatus efficiently and with proper care.

Electric Lights

These are dusted daily if they can be reached. Centre lights may be so high that they can be washed only periodically, and this is done by cleaners or by the electricians, who may be responsible for washing all electric light fittings.

When using a wet duster for cleaning electric lights or shades care should be taken to see that switches are first turned off. This precaution should also be taken when bulbs are being removed or replaced.

The best type of shade for large lights is the "hygienic" type, with no flutings or ridges to collect dust.

Metal Fittings

Brass and copper fittings, if not lacquered, are cleaned with metal polish; basin taps, chain and plugs require daily cleaning. Chromium plating and stainless steel have largely replaced brass and copper; these metals are much easier to keep clean as they only require washing with soapy water and finishing with a dry, soft cloth. Brass polish should never be used on chromium-plated articles.

Woodwork

Plain wood surfaces should be scrubbed along the way of the grain with soap and water, well rinsed with cold water and dried as completely as possible.

Treatment and Preparation Rooms

In most modern hospital wards provision is made for surgical dressings and other sterile procedures to be carried out in an annexe. Such provision is very desirable from the point of view of safe aseptic practice.

Adjacent to the treatment room two annexes are needed: one annexe is a "clean" preparation room where instruments and equipment are sterilized and trolleys prepared; the other annexe is a "dirty" utility room where used equipment is cleaned and the bin for soiled dressings is kept. It is most important that every possible step should be taken to prevent dust contamination of articles in the treatment and preparation areas, for example by keeping windows closed, reducing traffic as far as possible and providing adequate dust-proof storage cupboards for equipment. The boiling water sterilizer, steel bowls and other steel equipment should be maintained in good condition; in hard water areas daily cleaning with soap and steel wool or other abrasive may be needed. Glass shelves and trolleys should be washed with soap and water or dilute detergent solution. Trolley wheels need periodic cleaning and oiling.

The Ward Kitchen

Gas and electricity should be used with care. Great economy can be effected by immediately turning off when not required, and by not having a fiercer heat than is needed.

The cleaning of stoves and hot plates is usually the ward maid's work, but any milk or food spilt on the stove should be wiped up at once. The vitreous enamel finish for gas and electric cookers gives a surface which is easily cleaned.

Saucepans should be cleaned as soon as possible after use. Milk saucepans should be used for that purpose only, and filled with cold water before cleaning.

No soda must be used in the cleaning of aluminium ware.

Feeding cups require care in washing; the spouts should be cleaned with a bottle brush and then well rinsed.

The nurse is responsible also for seeing that all crockery and utensils are perfectly clean when patients' trays are set.

Crockery from infectious cases must be kept separate, washed and boiled after use. In some hospitals all ward crockery is boiled after every meal, and this is the usual practice in tuberculosis and infectious diseases hospitals.

Special feed and milk jugs must be inspected by the nurse before use. All special feeds must be covered and labelled.

Refrigerator cabinets should be washed thoroughly at regular intervals using, when necessary, warm water and soap to remove marks. The addition of baking soda (1 teaspoonful of bicarbonate of soda to 1 quart of water) to the washing water "freshens" the interior of the cabinet and counteracts food odours. Unless the type of refrigerator in use has an automatic defrosting mechanism, regular defrosting is necessary as a thick coating of frost on the freezing unit acts as an insulator and the temperature inside the cabinet will then tend to rise. Defrosting is carried out by turning off the current, or turning the control knob back to a point marked "defrost," removing the ice trays from the freezer unit, and either covering or removing the articles on the shelves. The melting ice collects in the drip tray under the freezer unit. Defrosting can be accelerated by placing a container of hot water inside the freezer unit. When the process is finished and the tray has been emptied and replaced, the interior of the cabinet is dried, the articles are replaced and the control knob is turned to give the required degree of coldness. Any food or liquid spilt on the refrigerator shelves should be wiped up immediately.

Hot dishes should be allowed to cool before being placed in the refrigerator.

Infants' feeds are kept in the refrigerator. Milk is usually delivered in bottles; it should be kept in the coolest part of the larder or in the refrigerator.

Larder shelves must be kept tidy and washed daily. All food must be covered.

Unwanted food, such as extra vegetables or an unwanted milk pudding, should be returned to the central kitchen, if they are not going to be used that day. For food refuse a "pig pail" is usually provided and the contents are sold for pig food. No tins, tea leaves, paper, egg shells or lemon or orange peel must be placed in this pail. All refuse bins must be kept covered.

When plates are stacked up ready for washing the bits

must be removed and all food waste put in the pig pail. A strainer or sink basket will help to prevent the waste pipe of the sink getting blocked with grease and tea leaves.

Any general repairs required, such as blocked waste pipes or dripping taps, should be reported at once.

Ward Bathrooms and Sanitary Annexes

Baths and lavatory basins are cleaned with soap and cleaning powder. Special care must be paid to the area under the taps, the overflow and the waste outlet. An old pair of forceps is useful for removing bits that tend to clog the waste pipe.

The washing bowls and mouth wash mugs are also cleaned with soap and cleaning powder and should be washed in hot soapy water containing 1–80 lysol, or boiled.

Dirty Dressing Pails. It is very desirable that soiled dressing bins and pails should be dealt with in a central station if staff, space and equipment for this can be provided. The containers are collected from the wards by porters, the contents burnt and the pails washed, disinfected by steam and returned clean to the wards. If the dressing pails have to be cleaned in the ward annexe they should be washed with a mop and disinfectant (*e.g.* crude phenol type of disinfectant 1–10), rinsed with boiling water and turned up to drain. When dry they may be lined with paper. Alternatively, the soiled dressings may be placed in paper containers (using forceps); these containers are then placed in the bins.

Bedpans and Urinals. These are flushed with cold water after use and then cleaned with a mop. Automatic bed-pan washers in which the bed-pans are enclosed for flushing with hot and cold water, are used in most hospitals. The use of this type of washer has the advantage of keeping the sluice room free from unpleasant odours and also reducing the handling of bed-pans by the nurses. The automatic bed-pan washer does not sterilize the utensils, and where this is necessary the best method is by boiling in a large tank sterilizer.

Sputum Mugs. Metal and enamel mugs are emptied and flushed (the sputum is weighed or measured first if necessary), and then boiled for five minutes. 1 fl. oz. sodium bicarbonate solution 1–160 is added before taking the sputum mug to the patient.   In some hospitals square tin sputum containers with cardboard linings are used.   The inner lining is removed and sawdust added to the sputum, which is then burned. Great care has to be taken when dealing with tuberculous sputum; cardboard containers which are disposed of by burning are generally used.   The containers should be collected by a porter specially allocated and instructed in this duty.   If the nursing staff have to handle the sputum containers of tuberculous patients, gloves, gown and mask should be worn.

Water Closets. The pan should be sprinkled with powder containing chlorinated soda and left for half an hour, it is then scrubbed with the lavatory brush and flushed.   The brush should be kept in an enamel holder with disinfectant such as Jeyes fluid 1–40 dilution.

Care of Bedsteads and Bedding

The usual hospital bedstead is made of enamelled iron. At one time black bedsteads were in general use but in recent years the wards have been brightened by the use of lighter colours and bedsteads are now frequently painted in cream or pastel colours or are given an aluminium finish.

Bedsteads should be dusted with a damp duster.   If possible they should be thoroughly washed once a week. The springs should be kept free from dust and rust; for this an oily rag is useful (see p. 55).

Any defective springs or broken wires should be reported at once, as the wire frame will sag and the bed is then uncomfortable; also the mattress or bedclothes may get torn.

Mattresses should be protected by the use of a short mackintosh (about 1 yard square) under the draw sheet, and where necessary by a long mackintosh completely covering the mattress under the bottom sheet or by a plastic mattress cover.   Pillows likely to be soiled by discharge or excreta should have mackintosh or plastic covers under the linen ones.

Bed Mackintoshes, Air Rings and Beds

These articles should be thoroughly scrubbed after use with warm water and soap.   If necessary, they may first be mopped with 1–20 phenol or 1–30 lysol solution.

They should be well rinsed and dried with a cloth, afterwards being hung up until completely dry.   They should not be placed on or near very hot radiators. Bed mackintoshes should not be folded; they are usually stored on rollers, or may be hung over rollers in a mackintosh cupboard.

Air rings and beds should be tested for leaks before being put away. A little air should be left in to keep the inner surfaces apart. They may be dusted with French chalk.

Rubber articles will perish if oil or greasy substances are allowed to remain in contact with them.

Ward Linen

The Medical Research Council's Memorandum on the control of cross infection in hospitals recommends that great care should be taken in the handling of soiled linen because contamination may occur from discharges and from the scattering of dust particles. The Council also recommends that nurses who are concerned in the care of patients and the conduct of sterile procedures should not sort and count soiled linen.

The Collection of Soiled Linen

A suitable method of collecting soiled linen from the bedside is the use of wheeled trolleys fitted with canvas or plastic bags which can be removed, tied and sent for sorting. Soiled linen should be removed from the ward as expeditiously as possible and sorting should be carried out away from the ward unit. Where the care of incontinent patients involves the frequent changing of heavily soiled linen a special bin should be provided and a "foul washing" machine is usually installed.

There is at present a trend towards centralization of all hospital stores, including linen supplies. In many hospitals the checking of both soiled and clean linen is carried out in a central department. It is very desirable that nurses should handle soiled linen as little as possible in order to avoid contamination of their hands and the possible risk of infecting patients, therefore the central counting of soiled linen has much to recommend it. An added advantage is that the nursing staff is relieved of a task which takes considerable time if checking is to be carried out efficiently. It is also usually claimed that losses of linen are reduced by centralization. Nevertheless the student nurse should understand the proper care of linen and the safeguards necessary to prevent unnecessary damage and loss.

Rules for the Care of Ward Linen

(1) Linen should be used only for the purposes for which it is intended.

(2) Linen should be kept as clean as possible Frequent laundering of very soiled linen wears out the articles.

(3) All articles should be plainly marked and should be carefully checked before sending to the laundry.

(4) Linen should be carefully checked when received from the laundry.

(5) Linen should be inspected before being put away and any repairs required should be done before it is used.

(6) Lending and borrowing should be avoided if possible in order to reduce the risk of losses.

(7) All badly soiled and stained linen should be dealt with immediately on removal from the bed.

Removal of Stains from Linen

Blood. Soak at once in cold water; when decolourized wash in warm soapy water. If the stain is thick and dried into the material, apply a bleaching agent, either peroxide of hydrogen or ammonia. Rinse well afterwards.

Ink. This should be treated at once by putting the article to soak in cold water or in milk; prolonged soaking, at least twenty-four hours, may be required. Rubbing a paste of salt and lemon juice on the stain and allowing the article to lie in the sun is another method which may be effective. Ball-pen ink stains can be removed by the application of methylated spirit.

Tea, Coffee and Cocoa Stains. Wash in cold water and then pour boiling water on the stain. If not completely removed, apply a bleaching agent and rinse well afterwards.

Fruit Stains. Rub with salt first and then treat as above.

Rust Marks. Salt and lemon juice and exposure to sunlight may be successful, but these marks are difficult to remove, especially if the linen has been laundered in the meantime.

Iodine. Apply ammonia, rinse and then wash.

Stains caused by drugs applied to the skin or excreted in the urine are often resistant to removal and may require special methods.

4

General Care of the Patient

GENERAL nursing care is a term that describes the essential function of the nurse which few if any of the other members of the "therapeutic team" perform except as a very occasional part of their function. It may be described as assisting the sick person in need of help for any reason in carrying out the ordinary functions of daily life, such as washing, dressing, moving, eating and elimination which the healthy adult performs with little thought or effort and as a matter of habit. Obviously the degree to which assistance is required must vary in every individual sick or dependent human being; unconscious patients, very ill patients, the very young and the very old may be quite unable to carry out any of the normal bodily functions without continual care and assistance from the nurse. In convalescence the nurse's skill may be exercised to the full in encouraging and promoting the patient's return to independence. The art of nursing is largely concerned in assessing and providing the degree of assistance necessary in a given situation. In this chapter and the two following ones some of the aspects of basic nursing are discussed and in describing methods used in carrying out certain procedures the statements are inevitably somewhat dogmatic. The nurse should always remember that modifications in practice often have to be made and the procedure adapted to suit the individual.

Sanitary Rounds

It is the usual practice to give bed-pans or urinals at definite times throughout the day to all patients confined to bed; *e.g.* the early morning, before the ward is opened after the morning cleaning, and after each meal time. Many patients will, of course, require attention at other than the routine times and this should always be given promptly.

The ward is closed to all but the nursing staff during the sanitary round. Privacy for the patient using the bed-pan should always be afforded, and where cubicle curtains are used in the wards this is easily and quickly provided, otherwise screens must be used.

The "Perfection" type of bed-pan is most comfortable for the patient, as it fits the contours of the body better than the round pattern. The materials used are porcelain, enamel ware and stainless steel. This last material has the advantage of being practically indestructible and will not chip or dent; the disadvantages are the high initial cost and the weight of the utensil. A rubber bed-pan may be used for incontinent patients, as it can be left in position without causing as much pressure as the hard rim of the usual type. Urinals are supplied in glass, enamel ware, polythene plastic and stainless steel.

The bed-pan should be warmed before giving it to the patient and heated racks are usually provided for this purpose in the sluice annexe. If a heated rack is not available the bed-pan should be warmed under the hot water tap, care being taken to see that it is not more than comfortably warm when given to the patient. Heated bed-pan trolleys may be used. The bed-pans are kept in the racks of the trolley, which is plugged into the electric power point and the heating is thermostatically controlled. The trolley is disconnected and wheeled into the ward for the sanitary round. An unheated trolley may be used for the collection of used bed-pans.

It is usual to cover the bed-pan or urinal when giving or removing it; for this purpose thick paper squares (paper towels) are very suitable as they can be discarded each time after use. Where trolleys are used for both clean and used bed-pans, no cover is usually required.

When the bed-pan is brought to the bedside the bedclothes should be turned down leaving the patient covered with a blanket. If an air-ring is used it should be removed before inserting the bed-pan. The patient who is allowed to help himself should be asked to pull his knees up, and the nurse will then assist him by placing her right arm under the lower part of the patient's back and then inserting the bed-pan with her left hand. When the patient has had his bowels open, toilet paper may be insufficient for cleansing purposes and good quality tow swabs, warm water, soap, dry tow or wool swabs, a receiver for soiled swabs and a towel will be needed. Tow or wool should not be flushed down the sluice but should be removed with forceps and placed in a bin provided for the purpose.

Patients are now often able to get up for washing and toilet purposes and the nurse should know which of these patients require some help. For patients unable to walk wheeled "lavatory chairs" are used. The seat of the chair has a space shaped to fit over the water closet pan and the patient can be wheeled from his bed to the toilet. A useful type of commode chair is one which also allows a bed-pan to be placed in position on a tray under the opening in the seat.

Patients who can attend to their own needs should be given washing water, soap and towel to wash their hands after using the bed-pan. After attending to the sanitary needs of a patient the nurse should wash her hands thoroughly. Hand basins should be provided near all toilets for both staff and patients so that the necessary washing of the hands can be carried out at once.

Bathing

(1) **In the Bathroom.** When the patient is allowed to go to the bathroom, the nurse should see that all requirements are there, including a dressing gown and slippers, that the windows are shut and the bathroom warm. The bath should be prepared at the correct temperature; 100° to 105°F. is the usual temperature for a hot cleansing bath.

Ward bathroom doors are not as a rule locked on the inside, but a screen may be put round the bath to give the patient a greater feeling of privacy. The nurse is responsible for seeing that the hands, feet and hair receive due attention.

(2) **In Bed.** *Requirements:*
   A large washing basin.
   A supply of hot water.
   Soap and two washing flannels.
   Two towels.
   A nail brush and nail scissors.
   Mouth wash, tooth brush and tooth paste.
   Surgical spirit, or a mixture of spirit and oil, and dusting powder may be needed.

A brush and comb. (Where necessary a small-toothed comb, a bowl of phenol lotion, 1–60, some wool swabs, a mackintosh cape and a receiver must be provided.)

Two bath blankets. If these cannot be kept for the patient's own use, a large bath towel should be provided and the patient's own bed blankets used.

The windows on either side of the patient should be closed and the bed screened or the curtains drawn. The hot-water bottle should be refilled and placed at his feet. The top of the bed is then stripped, leaving the patient covered with one blanket. If bath blankets are used, one should be rolled under the patient and the other used to cover him. The gown should be put to warm near the fire or on hot-water pipes.

The water used for washing should be as hot as the nurse's hand can comfortably bear and should be changed when it becomes cool or soiled. The patient's face should be washed first and, if allowed, he will probably like to do this for himself. The neck and ears are then washed and well dried. Each part should be washed quickly and thoroughly, though exposing the patient as little as possible. After the arms have been washed the hands should be well soaped and rinsed in the bowl. The chest and abdomen are washed next, paying special attention to the skin of the umbilicus in dirty or neglected patients. After washing the legs the bowl may be placed on the bed, and the feet well soaked and then rinsed in the bowl.

If the patient is able to help he is given a well-soaped flannel and allowed to wash the groins and between the legs, if not, this must be done for him.

When the patient is turned on his side to have his back washed a second nurse may be required to support him.

When the lower part of the back is being washed special care should be given to the cleanliness of the skin of the anal area and when washing the buttocks the nurse should carefully wash and dry the area between the legs while the patient is lying on his or her side.

When the bath is completed the blankets should be removed, the patient left covered with one of the bed blankets, his gown replaced and the bed re-made.

Necessary attention to the back and other pressure areas is given at the time of bathing and at regular intervals throughout the twenty-four hours. For details of this care see p. 36.

Care of the Mouth

If a patient is able to sit up in bed to clean his own teeth he should be supported in a comfortable position with a towel to protect his jacket and the sheet. He needs a tooth glass or metal mug containing tepid or hot water according to preference, tooth paste, brush and a large receiver or basin. Some patients like to use tooth picks or "dental stimulators" and most will like to finish the process with a pleasantly refreshing mouth wash. If the patient cannot sit up, he should be turned to his left side with the towel spread under his head and neck and the receiver on the towel conveniently placed for him to spit into.

A patient who is not able to assist himself should lie on his side as described above. The teeth are cleaned by brushing systematically with a moist tooth brush and the dentifrice, beginning with the outer surfaces of the front teeth, then with patient opening his mouth widely enough to allow the brush to be inserted between the inner surface of the cheek and the teeth; clean first the teeth on the right side and then on the left side and finally brush the inner surface of the teeth. The patient should be allowed to rinse freely during the process, and if he cannot raise his head sufficiently to use a tooth glass, an angled drinking tube should be provided. The state of the tongue and mouth should be noted during the tooth-cleaning process. False teeth must receive frequent attention, they should be scrubbed in clean warm water with a small brush, using bicarbonate of soda or a special dentifrice. The patient should be given a mouth wash after the dentures have been cleaned and replaced.

In acute illness the mouth requires frequent and careful attention. This is especially important in the case of patients who are on a limited fluid diet and regular two-hourly attention should be given. Neglect causes great discomfort and, in the case of a patient able to take little or nothing by mouth, may lead to the serious condition of parotitis (inflammation of the parotid glands). In the case of an unconscious patient the danger of inhaling material into the air passages must always be borne in mind and, in order to prevent this, the foot of the bed should be raised so that the patient's head is at a lower level than his trunk; suction may also be required in these cases.

A tray should be prepared with the following articles:

Wool swabs.

Catch forceps or small mouth sticks.

Two small gallipots containing glycerin of thymol, and hydrogen peroxide, or sodium bicarbonate or other suitable cleansing agents as may be preferred.

A mouth wash.

A kidney dish.

A receptacle for the dirty swabs.

A wood or metal spatula.

The teeth and gums should be carefully swabbed using several swabs wrapped round the forceps or sticks. All surfaces of the teeth and the crevices between the teeth should receive attention. The inner side of the cheeks and the tongue are cleansed in the same way. After this is completed the patient should rinse his mouth out with the mouth wash, if able to do so. The nurse should place a towel and the kidney dish under his chin and support his head.

Although the care of the patient's mouth is a most important nursing duty which should never be neglected it may be noted that severe infection of the mouth is comparatively seldom seen now in post-operative cases. This is due to the changed outlook on the feeding of patients after operation. Starvation or prolonged strict fluid diet are seldom prescribed and the importance of chewing as a natural cleansing agent for the tongue and mucous membrane of the mouth, with its stimulating effect on the flow of saliva and on the circulation, is well recognized.

Care of the Hair

The hair should be brushed and combed twice a day. Long hair is most comfortably dressed by braiding it in two plaits. Some hospital patients on admission require to have the head combed with a fine-toothed comb and then washed. This is usually ordered at the discretion of the ward sister.

Requirements:

Brush and comb and fine-toothed comb.

Bowl of 1–20 phenol, or Dettol 1–40, lotion.
Receiver.
Wool swabs.

When carrying out this treatment the nurse should stand behind the patient who will then not be able to watch the process.

The mackintosh cape should be placed round the patient's shoulders and the hair first brushed and combed free from tangles. Then dipping the small-toothed comb in the lotion, the nurse should take a small strand of hair and comb it through carefully, afterwards wiping the comb on a swab and inspecting the swab. This is continued until the hair has been carefully combed through.

A head which is found to be infested with lice or their eggs (nits) should be treated at once. Several methods are in use.

1. **Lethane Oil.** The infested head is treated by the application of an oil composed of 50 per cent. liquid paraffin and 50 per cent. Lethane 384 Special. Eight partings should be made in the hair, four on each side of the mid-line. The oil is then applied to the scalp from a teaspoon or a dropper and spread by massaging the scalp thoroughly. Following the application the hair should be combed daily to remove dead lice and nits but it should not be washed or brushed vigorously for the following eight days as the aim is to leave the oil on the scalp for sufficient time to kill the parasites. Lethane oil also kills nits.

2. **DDT Emulsion** (Suleo). This is applied in the same way as Lethane. The hair may be washed 48 hours after this application.

To wash the Hair of a Patient in Bed. *Requirements:*
Two mackintoshes and a mackintosh cape.
A shampoo lotion.
Two towels.
A basin.
A large jug of hot water.
A small jug, such as a pint measure.
A rubber hot-water bottle freshly filled, or a small radiant heat lamp or a hand electric hair drier.

The patient's gown should be slipped down below the armpits and the upper part of the chest covered with a blanket or warm bath towel, and the cape placed round the shoulders over this.

The top of the mattress may be turned under and should be covered with a mackintosh. The second mackintosh should cover the wire spring, and on this the bowl is placed. It is not possible to turn down an interior spring mattress but in this case the patient may be moved down the bed leaving a space at the top of the bed large enough to accommodate the washing bowl; two or three pillows placed under the patient's shoulders will support her while her head rests over the bowl. If the head of the bedstead can be removed the washing bowl can be placed on a chair.

The shampoo lotion should be well rubbed into the scalp, using the tips of the fingers. The hair should then be rinsed by pouring water on from the small jug and the shampooing process repeated. After a second rinsing the bowl is removed and the mattress replaced. The hair should be spread out on a towel with a mackintosh underneath and dried with a warm towel. The use of the hand radiant lamp or an electric hair drier will hasten the drying. If the hair is thick and long it should be combed out gently strand by strand when half dry to prevent it from becoming tangled. If the patient cannot lie down, a bed table may be placed behind her or in front, as is most conventient, and the bowl put on this.

If a patient's scalp is dry and full of dandruff and the hair cannot be washed frequently, the scalp should be rubbed with a mixture of surgical spirit and water followed by thorough brushing.

Care of the Nails

Finger nails should be kept short and trimmed to the shape of the finger. Toe nails should be cut straight across.

Plenty of soap and a soft nail brush should be used if the nails are dirty, and they should be cleaned after washing while the skin is soft. Olive oil may be applied before washing to loosen ingrained dirt in cases where the patient's hands or feet are very neglected.

Use of Hot-Water Bottles and Other Heating Appliances

Hot-water bottles are commonly used as a means of warming a bed in preparation for the reception of a patient, and some authorities consider that they should be used for this purpose only and should not be left in the bed with the patient. However, a well-protected rubber hot-water bottle can be a source of comfort to a patient, provided that he is fully conscious, able to appreciate heat and to move fairly freely in bed. Even under these conditions the nurse must appreciate that there is still a risk of burning the patient if the cover is insufficiently protected or if it leaks.

In some hospitals it is the practice to fill bottles from the hot-water supply tap, this water will be well below boiling point. Alternatively boiling water is poured into a jug from which the bottle is filled. It should be about two-thirds full, and after expelling the air the stopper is replaced and the bottle inverted and shaken to test for leaking. If this test is satisfactory, the bottle is dried and placed in the cover. The cover should be large enough to cover the entire bottle including the stopper, and preferably made of flannel. Some hospitals use two covers on each hot-water bottle.

The danger of placing hot-water bottles in the bed of a patient who is unconscious, paralysed or not able to appreciate sensations of heat or pressure is that the pressure of the bottle against the patient's skin can cause damage, even although the bottle may be properly protected and the temperature of the water it contains may not be hot enough to cause a burn unless associated with pressure.

Electrically heated pads and blankets are very useful for warming a bed ready for the reception of a new patient or a patient returning from the theatre.

The blanket should be placed flat in the bed over the bottom sheet and when switched on this should be indicated by a light. There is usually a waterproof covering to protect the interior of the blanket from moisture and in addition the blanket should have a clean cotton cover which can be changed for each patient. Electric blankets should not as a rule be left in an occupied bed and if for any reason this is ordered in a special case, it may be sandwiched between two woollen blankets.

Bedsores and Pressure Sores

Bedsores are ulcers which may occur in a patient confined to bed especially if his nutritional state is poor. In order to prevent their occurrence the nurse should clearly understand the conditions likely to lead to their formation.

Immediate Causes of a Bedsore

(1) *Pressure.* Where any bony prominence presses upon the bed the tissues lying between will have their blood supply reduced, and if this condition is allowed to persist the superficial tissues will die and the skin will break down, forming an ulcer.

(2) *Friction.* Friction from the bedclothes or from any cause will make the skin inflamed and sore, eventually leading to a breach of the skin.

(3) *Moisture.* The skin is made sodden and unhealthy by a continued moist condition.

Predisposing Causes. Certain patients are much more liable to the development of bedsores than others. Particular care must be taken in the following cases:

(1) Helpless or unconscious patients.
(2) Paralysed patients.
(3) Incontinent patients.
(4) Patients who are acutely ill, especially if toxæmia is marked.
(5) Very emaciated patients.
(6) Patients who are œdematous.

Prevention of Bedsores. Every effort should be made to prevent the occurrence of a bedsore as these ulcers are very slow to heal once they form. The encouragement of the circulation in the superficial tissues and the relief of pressure are the most important factors in the prevention of bedsores. When the area subjected to pressure is washed and dried the friction of the flannel and the towel and the gentle movement of the skin over the underlying tissues improves the flow of blood to the part and this is further helped by the relief of pressure when the patient is turned on to his side or lifted off the bed to change his position. In health the body seldom remains for long in one position, even during sleep, and when the patient is unable to change his own position the nursing staff must undertake this task for him at regular intervals. In the case of a paralysed patient it may be necessary for two nurses to turn him or to lift his back off the bed for a few moments every hour in order to relieve the pressure on the shoulder blades and sacrum.

In addition to the measures described above, routine treatment by massage of the part with the nurse's well-soaped hand, followed by rinsing and careful drying of the area, is given at four-hourly intervals to the sacral area, the shoulder blades, heels and any other parts subject to pressure in a bedridden patient. The massage may be followed by the application of surgical spirit, or a mixture of spirit and oil, followed by a light dusting with powder; some authorities consider that spirit and powder should not be used and that careful drying of the part is all that is needed.

If the skin shows redness, dark discoloration or bruising, this should be reported immediately and every effort must be made to prevent the skin from breaking.

Various aids can be used to relieve pressure and friction, such as an air ring, or air bed, a sorbo mattress, pads of wool or of sorbo rubber. Pads of wool bandaged on the knees, elbows and heels will prevent friction in restless or emaciated patients. A bed cradle will keep the weight of the clothes from the knees and toes. An alternating pressure pad is useful in providing regular and frequent redistribution of pressure areas, particularly where frequent moving of the patient or changing the position in bed is difficult or inadvisable, as for example in the case of certain injuries or very heavy patients. The pad, which is made of plastic material, is placed over the mattress and under the bottom sheet. The apparatus consists of a motor operating an air pump and a pneumatic pad containing air tubes. When the apparatus is working alternate sets of air tubes are inflated and deflated.

The bed should be kept free from crumbs and creases. Patched and darned sheets should not be put under the patient. Chipped enamel bedpans should not be used and the bedpan should not be left under the patient longer than is necessary. Great care should be exercised in inserting and removing the bedpan in order to avoid any abrasion of the skin.

The skin should always be carefully dried after washing. Incontinent patients require frequent attention to keep them clean and dry. Whenever the patient is found to be wet or soiled, the parts should be thoroughly washed and then smeared with a mixture of zinc ointment and castor oil, or a silicone barrier cream, to protect the skin. Damp or

3

soiled bedclothes or gown should be immediately replaced by clean dry ones.

Sores may also occur from the pressure of a splint or plaster. Any complaint of pain or of a burning sensation should be reported at once. If the pressure is not relieved without delay, the part will become insensitive; and although the patient will no longer complain of pain, a large sore may form which will be very difficult to heal.

Treatment of Bedsores. If a bedsore or pressure sore does occur the treatment will depend upon the size and state of the ulcer. Large sloughing sores may require fomentations or charcoal poultices to aid in the separation of the sloughs, but the particular dressing to be used will be ordered by the doctor.

Silicone cream or gentian violet paint, 1 per cent., may be used. Shortwave treatment may be ordered, which will be carried out by the physiotherapist.

MOVING AND SUPPORTING THE PATIENT

Moving the patient is an art and, as in every art, an intelligent understanding of the underlying principles makes it comparatively simple. The basis of success is the application of the knowledge of anatomy and physiology at each stage in the different methods used.

The illustrations on the following pages show the correct methods of lifting the patient by hand and with the aid of a mechanical hoist, and also how to turn the patient, which is the best method of moving the patient if a small movement only is needed. A mechanical hoist can often be of great assistance to the nursing staff and enable a heavy helpless patient to be moved with comfort and safety. One type of patient lifter is supplied with a stretcher attachment for lifting a patient in a prone position and an attachment for lifting in the sitting position. (See Figs. 9 and 10.)

Lifting the Patient

In lifting, the position of the nurses' hands with regard to the skeleton is of great importance both for raising the patient satisfactorily from the bed and avoiding undue strain on the lifters. With the correct technique a heavy patient can be readily lifted without any effort on his part. It is also important that the two nurses work together smoothly, one being in charge and responsible for giving instructions to the patient. As many patients who require lifting are already sitting up in bed with the knee flexed, there is often a far more obvious hollow under the knees than at the gluteal fold. If the hands are slipped under the knees, the lift will be difficult if not impossible. If the hands are high up in the gluteal fold, a perfect lift becomes an easy matter.

The patient should first be told to cross his hands on the chest; if he is to be lifted up in the bed, his head should be flexed so that his chin rests on his sternum. If he is being raised for care of the back or bedmaking, his head should rest back on his pillows.

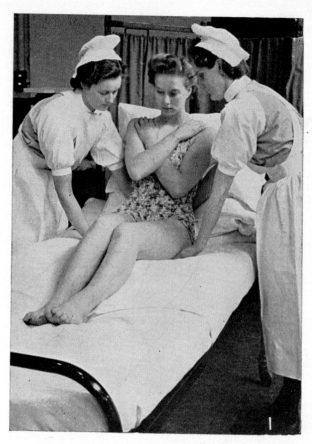

FIG. 1.—LIFTING A PATIENT.   I.

The patient is first raised from the pillows.   Each nurse places the arm nearest the head of the bed behind the small of the patient's back, one grasping the other firmly round the wrist.   The nurses' lower hands are slipped under the patient in the natural hollow at the junction of the thigh and buttock. One nurse again grasps the other's wrist firmly.   It is better for each nurse to grip with one hand and be gripped with the other.

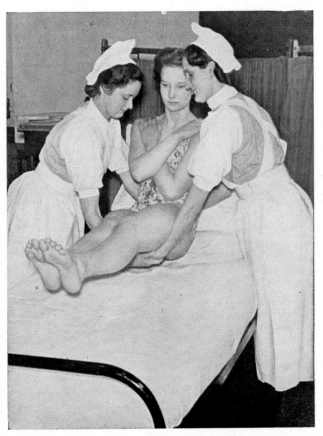

FIG. 2.—LIFTING A PATIENT. II.

The nurses now press their knees against the bed and lift the patient, using the muscles of the hip and knee, which are so much stronger than those of the shoulder and elbow. The patient is easily lifted clear of the bed for bedmaking, care of the back, or the insertion of the bedpan. Note how the patient is, as it were sitting on the lower wrists of the nurses who are lifting her.

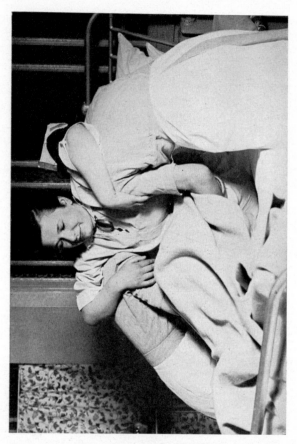

FIG. 3.—AN ALTERNATIVE METHOD OF LIFTING A PATIENT.

Both nurses face the head of the bed. The nurse on the left side of the patient places her left shoulder as a crutch under the patient's axilla. She passes her left arm under the upper part of the patient's thighs and grasps the right wrist of the nurse on the opposite side of the bed whose right shoulder under the patient's right axilla acts as a crutch on that side.

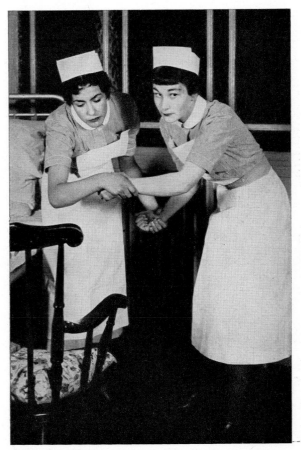

Fig. 4.—Carrying a Patient from a Bed to a Chair. I.

This is the correct position for the nurses' arms when lifting the patient from the bed to a chair.

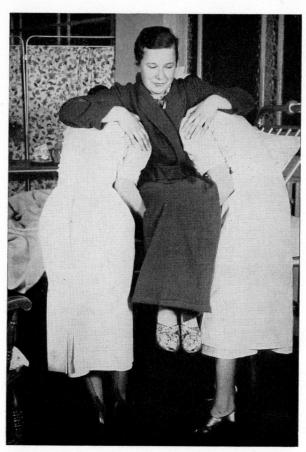

Fig. 5.—Carrying a Patient from a Bed to a Chair. II.

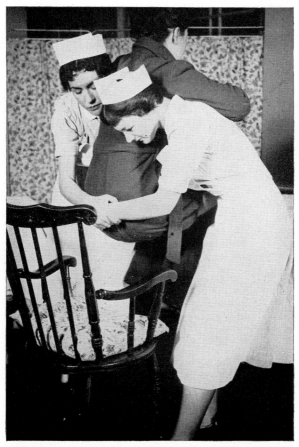

FIG. 6.—CARRYING A PATIENT FROM A BED TO A CHAIR. III.

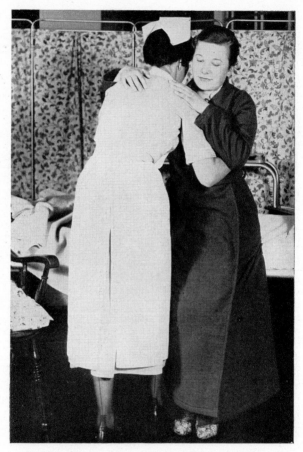

Fig. 7.—Moving a Patient from a Bed to a Chair.   I.

This method of supporting a patient from her bed to a chair is used when she is unable to take any weight on the shoulders.

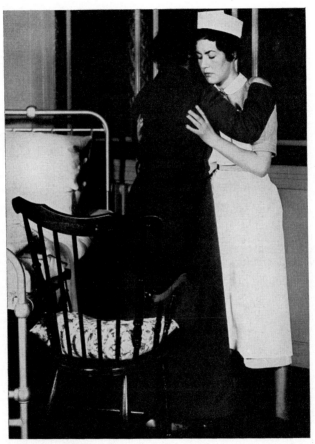

FIG. 8.—MOVING A PATIENT FROM A BED TO A CHAIR. II.

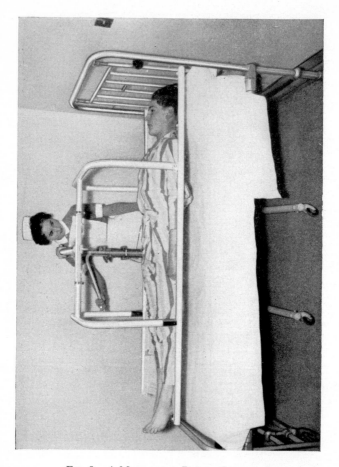

Fig. 9.—A Mechanical Patient Lifter.   I.

The patient being lifted easily from the bed by means of the hydraulic pump.

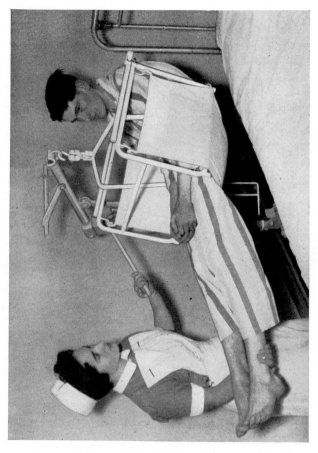

Fig. 10.—A Mechanical Patient Lifter. II.

The patient is raised and swung clear of the bed for transportation.

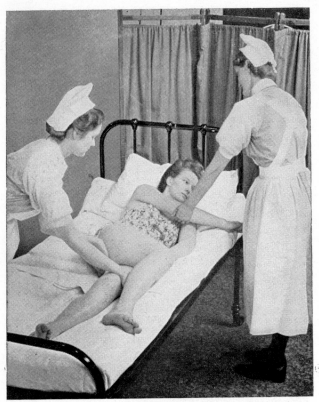

FIG. 11.—TURNING THE PATIENT. I.

Begin by placing the limbs in the correct position. First move the arm towards which the patient will move well away from the body. Then move the limbs on the opposite side of the body across the trunk towards the side on to which the patient is to be rolled, bending the knee at the same time. The weight of the limbs causes the trunk to be tilted in the required direction before any further step is taken. The nurses' hands can then readily be slipped well under the shoulder and pelvic girdles, in preparation for turning the patient.

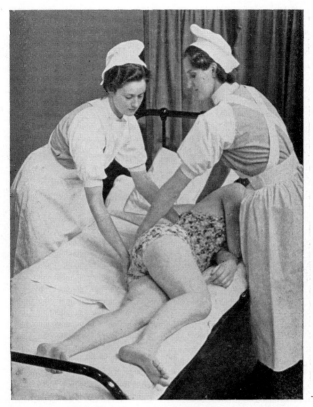

FIG. 12.—TURNING THE PATIENT. II.

Next the nurses slip their hands under the shoulder and pelvis and, pressing their knees against the bed, gently roll the patient over. The bulk of the work is done by the nurse towards whom the patient is turning; she leans back, working mainly with the muscles of the knee, hip and lower part of the back, with little active movement of the shoulders and arms.

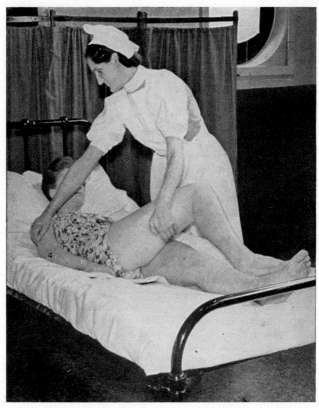

FIG. 13.—TURNING THE PATIENT. III.

Wrong method. The right leg and arm have not been brought across the trunk as the first step in rolling the patient. The nurse cannot get her hand satisfactorily under either the shoulder or pelvic girdles. Her right hand does not give her a good grip likely to give the patient confidence. Her left hand is under the thigh instead of the pelvis. The patient has been told not to exert herself at all, and therefore the nurse has not been able to move the shoulders satisfactorily and has merely drawn the thigh across the trunk instead of moving the pelvis.

5

Admission and Discharge of Patients: Last Offices

Admission of a Patient

WHEN a patient who has been on the list for admission arrives at the ward, he should be given a chair while the necessary forms are completed and the information required is obtained. First impressions are apt to be very lasting; the nurse should remember this and not be brusque or hurried in her manner.

The particulars generally required from the patient or his relatives are as follows:

Name and address.

Age.

If married or single, widow or widower.

Occupation—in the case of a child the father's occupation.

Religion.

The address of the nearest relative (if not the same as the patient's address) and the telephone number, or the telephone number of a neighbour or friend willing to take a message.

The name of the physician or surgeon in charge of the case.

The name and address of the patient's general practitioner.

If the patient is a child, it is important to obtain full particulars, including the child's previous medical history, from the parents before they leave the ward. They should also sign a form giving permission for an operation to be performed, or for an anæsthetic to be given if it is at all likely that these procedures will be required.

The relatives should receive a list of articles required by the patient, a list of articles that may be brought in and a

4+

permit for visiting at the stated times. If the patient is seriously ill a special visiting permit is usually given, and the relatives should be told when to enquire or visit again.

The temperature and the pulse and respiration rates should be taken and written down.

Unless contra-indicated, a bath is prepared and the patient taken to the bathroom.

The condition of the patient's skin, the presence of any sores, bruises or scars, and the state of general cleanliness including the hair, should be reported to the ward sister.

Many patients are allowed to be up for part of the day and most will therefore require suitable indoor clothing. The provision of individual wardrobes is very desirable, but if patients' clothes are stored in a kit-room there should be a shelf and hanging space for each patient. The clothing of dirty and neglected patients may be infested with fleas or lice and will need to be disinfected. This clothing should be placed in a canvas bag and labelled. The usual methods of disinfection used are steam under pressure or formalin vapour in an airtight chamber.

If the patient is unable to go to the bath, he should be bathed in bed as soon as possible.

Admission of an Emergency Case. When a message is received that such a case is to be admitted, the nurse taking the message should, if possible, find out what is the matter with the patient, so that any special requirements can be prepared.

It is important to have a warm bed ready for the patient, and the bed is prepared as described on p. 63.

If his condition permits he is given a bath in bed.

Care of Valuables. Any large sums of money in the patients' possession or articles of value should be reported to the ward sister, so that they may be locked up. In many hospitals they are taken to a safe and the patient is given a receipted list.

Any drugs in the patient's possession should be given to the ward sister, who will keep them for the doctor's inspection.

Discharge of a Patient

When a patient is about to be discharged, the nurse

should ascertain that the patient has ready all the necessary clothing. Dressings, bandages or splints should be freshly applied immediately before the patient leaves the hospital. Any instructions regarding future attendance at the hospital or treatment which is to be carried out at home must be fully and carefully explained to the patient or his relatives. Should there be any criticism of the patient's treatment, or any question about his belongings, the nurse should at once report this to the ward sister, so that the matter can be dealt with before the patient leaves the hospital.

The patient is usually given a discharge form which has to be given to the porter on duty at the hospital entrance.

After the patient has been discharged the mattress and pillows may be disinfected; if this is not necessary, they are removed from the ward, well brushed and aired and, if possible, exposed to sunlight.

The bedstead is thoroughly washed and cleaned. Turpentine or paraffin are useful cleaning agents, as they will not rust the wire springs.

The bedside locker should be thoroughly washed, paying particular attention to the drawers and cupboard.

Last Offices

The fact that death has taken place must be certified by the doctor or the ward sister. The relatives should be left alone at the bedside for a few moments. Before leaving the hospital they should be interviewed by the doctor or the sister and also told when to return for the death certificate.

Notification of death is usually sent at once to the Matron's office, the Secretary's office and the Porter's lodge.

Any particular wish on the part of the relatives should receive sympathetic attention. If they have had a long and anxious time at the bedside, or if the death of the patient has been a sudden shock, the nurse should make sure that they are fit to leave the hospital. A quiet room in which to rest for a short time and a cup of tea or coffee should be offered.

When the relatives have left the bedside the top clothes are removed from the bed, leaving one sheet to cover the body, and the bottom sheet, draw sheet and mackintosh under the body.

Air rings, hot-water bottles, cradles and pillows should

be removed. The gown should be removed and also any jewellery, unless the relatives have expressed a wish that an article, such as a wedding ring, should remain. Their wishes regarding false teeth should also be ascertained. The eyes should be closed and small pledgets of damp cotton wool may be placed on the lids to keep them closed.

The mouth should be cleaned and then closed. A jaw bandage is often applied, but this may cause discoloration if tight, and a thick pad or small pillow under the jaw may be used instead.

The body should be placed perfectly straight in the bed with the feet together and the arms at the side. One pillow may be left under the head.

The body is then covered with the sheet and left for one hour.

At the end of this time the following articles will be required for completing the last offices.

A gown and clean sheets. These are usually special articles put aside for this purpose.

A washing bowl with warm water, soap, flannel and towels.

Brush and comb; if necessary a small-toothed comb.

Cotton wool.

Dissecting forceps, scissors and sinus or Spencer Wells forceps.

If there is a dressing, a bowl of phenol or chloroxylenol lotion 1–40, white lint, jaconet, bandages and a needle and cotton will be required.

Receiver or dirty-dressing bin for soiled swabs and soiled dressings.

A name card on which is written the patient's name, the time of death and the ward, and tape for tying the card to the wrist.

The body should be washed all over, using plenty of soap; the nails should be cleaned and cut short.

The rectum (and in the case of a female patient the vagina also if necessary) is plugged, using cotton wool.

Any dressings are removed, tubes are taken out and a phenol or chloroxylenol compress is applied. Bandages should be fastened with a small strip of adhesive tape. Safety pins should not be used for this purpose as a serious infection may result if the nurse pricks her finger.

The hair should be brushed and arranged neatly; if it is

long, it should be plaited and tied with white tape or a ribbon.

The gown should be put on with the opening down the back, the eye pads and jaw bandage are removed.

The name card should then be attached to the wrist and the body wrapped in the mortuary sheet.

The whole procedure should be carried out quietly and the bed should be well screened. It is important that all articles should be collected beforehand, so that the nurses do not need to move the screen at all until the procedure is finished.

The body should be taken from the ward as soon as possible.

All linen and blankets are sent to the laundry and the bedding should be fumigated, mackintoshes scrubbed, using a disinfectant such as Izal 1–40 solution.

The bedstead and locker should also be well washed and disinfected.

After drying the wire spring and polishing the enamel parts of the bedstead, fresh bedding and linen will be required to make up the bed once more.

All utensils used during the patient's illness and the articles used for the laying out should either be disinfected or boiled. Anything belonging to the patient, no matter how small in value, must be carefully kept. Any important or valuable articles such as jewellery, money, letters or documents, should be made into a separate parcel and given into the charge of the ward sister. Clothes and any articles of food should be made up into two separate parcels clearly marked with the name and bed number and a list of the articles enclosed. These are returned to the relatives who are usually asked to sign a receipt for the articles.

Screens should be left round the bed until it has been freshly made up and everything returned to its normal appearance.

6

Bed-making: General and Special

Bedding

THE type of mattress which has for many years been in general use in hospital wards is the hair-filled mattress. It is resilient, hard-wearing and relatively non-absorbent, and the introduction of interior springing in this type of mattress recently has greatly enhanced its comfort. A washable cotton cover should be used. Foam rubber mattresses are very suitable for some patients, they are buoyant as the interior consists of sponge rubber intersected with air spaces. They are easily cleaned and there is no need to use a long mackintosh; for these reasons the rubber mattress is particularly useful in the nursing of helpless and incontinent patients.

Pillows. Soft pillows are filled with feathers; firm pillows used for support or for a foundation are filled with hair.

Blankets. Best white wool, which is light and warm, is commonly used for top blankets, but this material has the disadvantage of becoming "felted" and thickened by constant washing. Recently Acrilan, a "man-made" fabric, which is less affected by laundering, and cotton cellular blankets, which can be boiled, have been introduced. Old thin blankets or flannelette may be used as under blankets, or next to the patient.

Counterpanes. These should be light in weight and light in colour, and able to withstand frequent washing.

Sheets and pillow cases are made of cotton, cotton and linen "union" or of linen. Linen looks nice and lasts well, but is expensive in the first place and some patients find it cold.

Draw sheets are made of twill cotton sheeting, which is warm and absorbent. They should be 2 yards wide (1 yard

when doubled) and $2\frac{1}{2}$ yards long—*i.e.* long enough to pull
through completely.

General Principles of Bed-making

The comfort or discomfort of the sick person largely
depends on the bed in which he is lying, its freshness, free-
dom from creases and crumbs and the proper arrangement
of pillows to give support where needed. The prime aim
in making the bed is to make the patient comfortable. It
is also desirable that the appearance of the bed shall be neat
and clean. Disorder and a lack of freshness react un-
favourably on the sick person.

All articles required should be collected before beginning
to strip the bed.

Two nurses should work smoothly together, avoiding
unnecessary steps, jarring the bed or jerky movements of
the mattress and patient.

The patient must not be exposed during the procedure.

Sufficient help must be available when necessary to move
the patient without danger to him and without causing pain.

The actual procedure varies somewhat in different training schools, and it is only possible to indicate the general
methods employed for various types of bed.

To make up an Unoccupied Bed. Collect the blankets,
sheets, pillow cases and mackintosh and place them on a
chair at the foot of the bed in the order in which they will
be required.

See that the mattress is pulled well up to the bed head.
Spread the under blanket over the mattress. Next spread
out the bottom sheet, allowing sufficient to tuck in firmly at
the foot. Tuck in the sides and the end.

Place the short mackintosh in position across the bed,
usually about 18 inches from the head. The draw sheet
must be wide enough to cover the mackintosh completely.
Tuck in about 1 foot of the draw sheet at one side; at the
other side the long end of the draw sheet is pleated or rolled
and tucked as smoothly and evenly as possible under the
mattress.

Spread out the top sheet, allow about 20 inches at the
top, and fold back or tuck in at the foot. Tuck in the sides.

Spread the blankets out, making sure that they will come
high enough up to cover the patient's shoulders. Tuck in

the blankets at the sides and then the foot; fold the top corners diagonally.

Spread out the counterpane, tuck in the bottom edge, fold the sheet back over the top and finish at the foot end by mitring the corners.

Pile the pillows at the head of the bed with the closed ends of the pillows facing the ward doors.

If the bed is made up ready for the immediate admission of a patient, the top clothes should be left untucked at one side.

To make an Occupied Bed. It is impossible to give any exact instructions as to which patients may be moved by rolling from side to side and which patients should be lifted, as opinions vary in different hospitals and also change from time to time. As a general rule in surgical cases most patients are allowed and encouraged to move about freely from the first day after operation. In the medical ward patients suffering from congestive heart failure, pneumonia and pleurisy are as a rule nursed sitting up and are lifted for bed-making and sheet-changing.

(1) *If the patient can get up* he should sit at the bedside wrapped in a blanket. The mattress can then be turned and the wire spring dusted as required.

(2) *To make a bed when the patient cannot get out, but may be allowed to turn from side to side:*

Place a chair at the foot of the bed.

Strip the counterpane, folding it loosely over the chair.

Strip the blankets separately, folding in the same way, but leaving one covering the patient.

Draw the top sheet down towards the feet, leaving the patient covered with the blanket when the sheet is removed.

Remove all but one of the pillows.

Pull up the mattress if it has slipped away from the head of the bed and dust the bed frame.

Untuck the under clothes, lift the patient's feet, brush out crumbs, straighten the under blanket and sheet.

Find out which side of the bed has the short end of the draw sheet. Roll the patient over towards this side. The nurse on that side of the bed places her hands one under his shoulders and the other under the buttocks and rolls the patient towards her (see pp. 50–52). He must be supported while on his side and a pillow placed under his head.

Straighten the under blanket and sheet on that side, removing any crumbs and tucking the sheet very firmly under the mattress.

Tuck in about 1 foot of draw sheet and gather the remainder into a roll against the patient's back.

Roll the patient right over on to his other side, supporting him as before. See that he is well covered by the blanket while being turned.

Straighten and tuck in the under blanket and sheet on the opposite side; unroll the draw sheet and tuck it in.

Roll the patient on to his back and then lift him forward with a nurse's hand under each axilla; then one nurse will support him while the other nurse shakes up the pillows and replaces them.

If the patient has slipped down in the bed, lift him up towards the head. The nurses grasp hands under the patient's shoulders and thighs, directing him to let his head flex on his chest while they lift him (see p. 40).

Another method of lifting a patient either in bed or from his bed to a chair is also illustrated on pp. 42-47. This method may sound somewhat complicated in description but reference to the photographs will make the principle clear, in effect the nurses' shoulders act as crutches. Both nurses face towards the head of the bed; the nurse standing on the patient's left side places her shoulder under his axilla and grasps the wrist of the second nurse, who is using her right shoulder as a crutch under the patient's axilla in the same way. As they lift together the patient is moved with ease and comfort.

Spread out the top sheet, remove the blanket covering the patient and complete the top of the bed.

(3) *If the patient is sitting upright and may not be rolled from side to side:*

Strip the bed, leaving the patient covered with one blanket. Untuck the sides of the bottom sheet. Lift his legs, brush out the bottom of the bed and straighten the bedclothes. Lift the patient to the foot of the bed, where he is supported by one nurse while the other makes the top part of the bed, shakes up and replaces the pillows.

Lift the patient back and finish the bed as before.

An alternative method that is often practicable, except in cases where the patient is so large that sufficient space is

4*

not available, is to lift the patient over to one side of the
bed while making the opposite side.

If neither of these methods is suitable then three nurses will
be required. When the top bedclothes have been removed,
two nurses lift the patient, while the third straightens and
tucks in the under blanket, bottom sheet and mackintosh,
pulling through the draw sheet.

To change the Under Sheet. (1) If the patient may be
turned on to his side the clean sheet should be rolled or
pleated lengthways.

Strip the top of the bed leaving one blanket to cover the
patient and turn him to one side. Roll the soiled under
sheet with the draw sheet and mackintosh up to the patient's
back.

Place the clean sheet in position along the side of the bed,
tucking it in and then bringing the roll up to that of the
soiled sheet.

Turn the patient over to the opposite side, remove the
soiled sheet, spread out the clean one and unroll the mackintosh and draw sheet. Complete the bed in the usual way.

(2) If the patient is not allowed to turn, the sheet should
be prepared by rolling it across the width instead of the
length, and it is put in from the top instead of from the side.

Untuck the soiled sheet at the head of the bed and roll
it down as far as possible.

Tuck in the clean sheet and bring the roll down to that
of the soiled sheet.

Raise the patient and remove the draw sheet and mackintosh; pull down the soiled sheet and the clean one.

Raise the patient's legs, removing the soiled sheet and
bringing down the clean one.

Lift the patient once more to replace the mackintosh and
draw sheet. If the patient is very heavy or helpless, two nurses
will be required to lift him while a third removes the draw
sheet and pulls down the soiled and the clean under sheets.

In some cases it is permissible to lift the patient down to
the foot of the bed after stripping the top clothes. One
nurse should support him while the other attends to the top
of the bed. He is lifted back when the draw sheet and
mackintosh have been replaced.

The changing of the bottom sheet may be done from the
foot of the bed towards the head. In some instances, *e.g.*

a patient with a fracture of the lower limb, this may be the most convenient method.

Cots. Cots for infants and toddlers are made in much the same way as beds for adult patients, but the counterpane will be tucked in under the mattress at the side instead of hanging down, as is the usual practice in making a bed. The child can usually be removed from the cot and held comfortably by a nurse sitting at the cot side while it is being made. The toddler is likely to spend more of his day sitting on his bed clothes than under them, and therefore in cold weather care must be taken to see that he is sufficiently warmly clad. The cot side must be pulled up in position and safely fastened before the nurses leave the cot side.

To change the Mattress of a Bedridden Patient. The easiest method is to make up another bed as far as the draw sheet and mackintosh, bring it alongside the patient's bed and then lift him on to the fresh bed. Alternatively a mechanical hoist may be used while the mattress is changed.

Special Beds

(1) **To prepare a Bed for an Emergency Admission.** In most cases the bed is prepared by placing hot-water bottles or an electric blanket in the bed and leaving the top bed clothes untucked at one side so that they can readily be turned back. If a patient is to be received fully clothed, as for example following a street accident, the bottom sheet should be protected by covering it with a long mackintosh and an old blanket or rug, rugs should also be provided to cover the patient.

(2) **To prepare a Bed for a Patient returning from the Operating Theatre.** The bed is first stripped, the frame dusted with a damp duster and clean linen put on the bottom of the bed. The top bed clothes are made up but left loose so that they may easily be rolled back when the patient returns from the theatre.

Two hot-water bottles covered with a folded blanket, or an electric blanket, are placed in the bed under the top bed clothes. The pillows are left at the side of the bed.

If the vomit bowl, tongue forceps, gag, swab holder and mops are not on the theatre trolley with the patient, these should be placed ready on the locker at the bedside.

Blocks should be in readiness to raise the foot of the bed.

If hypothermia (lowering of the body temperature) is used in anæsthesia the bed is not heated and the patient is at first covered with a sheet only.

(3) **Bed for a Tonsillectomy Case.** A mackintosh and towel are required to place under the head. Ice and mops must be ready at the bedside. The patient is placed in the semi-prone position on return from the theatre.

(4) **Beds for Abdominal or Thoracic Operation Cases.** The upright position with the knees flexed, known as Fowler's position, was at one time in general use for abdominal operation cases when the patient had recovered from the anæsthetic and from post-operative shock.

In recent years, however, with the increasing emphasis on the importance of early movement following operations, a modified "sitting up" position is commonly employed following abdominal and thoracic operations.

In order to support the patient in the *sitting position* as many as six pillows may be needed. The two under pillows may be firm ones, the rest should be feather. The pillows are piled one above the other, supporting the patient's back, and then one soft one is placed well down in the small of the back and a small soft pillow arranged to support the head. Alternatively support may be given by an adjustable bed-rest and three pillows, see fig. 14.

Raising the foot of the bed by blocks or a bed elevator is necessary in order to prevent the patient from slipping down the bed; a support for the patient's feet, such as a large covered sandbag or a padded board and a cradle to take the weight of the bedclothes off the feet will also be required.

(5) **Bed for a Patient with Traction applied to a Fracture of the Lower Limb.** The bed is made up with fracture boards under the mattress. An air ring will be required.

The upper part of the bed is made in two sections.

Top. Spread the sheet over the bed, and then a blanket with bottom edge to bottom edge of the sheet. Both together are folded in half, bottom to top and the top edge of sheet turned out in the usual way.

Bottom. Spread out a blanket with the bottom edge to the edge of the bedstead, turn over at the top where the gap between the sections will be needed. A second sheet may be used under the blanket at the lower half of the bed.

Tuck the quilt in at the foot in the usual way and fold over the top edge to correspond with fold of blanket.

(6) **Bed for a Patient whose Leg has been Amputated.** A divided bed similar to that described above may be used for the first forty-eight hours after operation for a patient who has had an amputation of the leg, in order that the dressing on the stump may be easily inspected without disturbing the patient. Many authorities, however, consider this practice unnecessary and undesirable, and the top bedclothes are then tucked in at the foot in the usual manner. A large cradle will be needed, also two sandbags and a cloth or roller towel to steady the stump. In the days when many amputations were undertaken for cases of severe septic infection, a tourniquet was usually kept on the bedstead in readiness for any occurrence of secondary hæmorrhage. This type of case is now seldom seen and moreover the use of a tourniquet is regarded with disfavour by many surgeons.

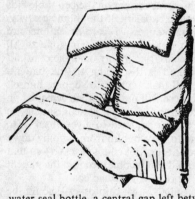

Two pillows on end are placed against the head rest and a third placed across them to support the head and shoulders. The rest and three pillows are a comfortable support and more economical in pillows and linen than are pillows only. In the bed illustrated, for a patient with a drainage tube in the thoracic cavity connected with a water seal bottle, a central gap left between the pillows prevents kinking or obstruction of the tube.

FIG. 14.—BED PREPARED WITH A BED REST AND THREE PILLOWS TO SUPPORT A PATIENT IN THE SITTING POSITION.

(7) **Beds for Patients suffering from Acute Rheumatism or Renal Disease.** It is not now the usual practice to nurse these patients between blankets, but a thin blanket or a flannelette sheet may be placed next to the patient under the top sheet. A cradle may be needed to take the weight of the

bed clothes off the painful joints or œdematous limbs and an air ring may be required.

(8) **Beds for Cardiac Cases.** In cases of acute carditis which often accompanies acute rheumatism the patient lies flat unless he is short of breath. A patient suffering from congestive heart failure is nursed sitting up, as he can then breathe more easily. If the condition is severe, the patient may not be able to breathe unless sitting upright and leaning forward with his arms supported on a bed table.

Additional requirements are as many pillows as may be necessary; a bed rest, an air ring and a light blanket.

The bed is made up with the draw sheet and mackintosh nearer the head of the bed than usual.

The light blanket is placed next to the patient.

A bed rest helps to support the patient and the pillows are arranged in an armchair fashion.

A bed table, with a soft pillow on it, placed over the bed allows the patient to lean forward for a change of position, and the wide spread of his arms resting on the bed table aids respiration by increasing the capacity of the thoracic cavity.

Patients suffering from congestive cardiac failure are particularly liable to slip down in the bed in spite of all efforts to maintain the necessary support, and the constant moving and lifting required is disturbing to the patient. In addition the patient will make efforts to support himself or to move himself and these will make further demands on an already failing circulation. Such a patient should be nursed in a bed which can be adjusted to give a back rest, and raised at the foot end to prevent him from slipping down the bed, and also dropped at the foot end if necessary so that drainage of œdematous fluid can be obtained and the patient given the additional comfort of a "cardiac chair".

(9) **Plaster of Paris Splints.** Mackintoshes should be put over the bottom sheet under the plaster until it is dry.

A bed cradle is required and the top clothes should be turned back at the bottom to allow free circulation of air.

A blanket next to the patient will keep him from getting chilled.

A large plaster applied to the leg or hip is likely to be very heavy, and the limb may be slung to a Balkan beam when the plaster has set.

(10) **Tent Bed.** This is used in conjunction with a steam

kettle in respiratory diseases, where it is desired to have a warm moist atmosphere round the patient.

A special frame is attached to the corners of the bedstead and supports a canopy and the tent sides. The tent may only surround the top half of the bed; if a complete tent is used, then an opening is left at one side. If the special frame is not available, screen frames may be used over which sheets are arranged.

Air Rings or Pillows

The square pillow is often more comfortable than the ring, which has a rather hard edge, although the ring is still in common use. A bicycle pump or bellows is needed to inflate air rings, air pillows and beds. Care should be taken to see that these are not inflated to a degree where they become hard and unyielding instead of soft and comfortable for the patient. Square pillows of sponge rubber may be preferred to air pillows. All rubber rings and pillows should be covered with a cotton case before being placed under the patient.

Prevention of "Foot Drop"

Any patient confined to bed may develop the condition known as "foot drop," but it is more likely to occur in patients who are paralysed and in patients who suffer a long debilitating illness. The muscles that plantar flex the foot exert more pull than the weaker muscles that dorsiflex the ankle joint, consequently when the patient eventually leaves his bed and should be starting to walk his progress is greatly hampered by foot deformity and by stiffness of the ankle joints. It is part of the nurse's duty to endeavour to prevent the occurrence of foot drop in three ways: (i) by supporting the feet at a right angle to the legs by means of a firm pillow padding a board or by the use of a sandbag, (ii) by ensuring that the top bedclothes are never tightly tucked over the patient's feet, a bed-cradle is needed to take the weight of the bedclothes off the feet of a helpless patient, (iii) by encouraging the patient to move his legs and to dorsiflex the ankle joints at regular intervals throughout the day, or by passively exercising the legs if the patient is unable to move them himself.

7

Observation and Recording of Temperature, Respiration, Pulse and Blood Pressure

Temperature

TEMPERATURE is the state of warmth or coldness of a substance or body compared with a standard. The thermometer is the instrument used to register temperature, based on the principle that all matter expands on heating and contracts on cooling.

Mercury is a convenient liquid to use for most thermometers, as it expands readily with a small change of temperature, readily takes the temperature of the body with which it is in contact and gives a level which is easily read.

Thermometer Scales. Whatever scale is used the fixed points are the same: the boiling point and freezing point of water at normal atmospheric pressure. On the Fahrenheit scale, which is the one principally used in this country, the boiling point of water is 212° and the freezing point 32° (180° between these two points). On the Centigrade scale, used in most European countries, the fixed points are 100° and 0°; there are therefore 100° between these two points. The Réaumur scale is used in some continental countries; on this scale the boiling point of water is 80° and the freezing point 0°. (For conversion of Centigrade and Fahrenheit scales, see p. 119.)

The Clinical Thermometer. This thermometer is graduated from 90° to 114° F.; it is made of thick-walled glass tubing with a narrow bore. A constriction above the bulb prevents the mercury dropping, when the thermometer is removed from contact with the patient, until it is reset by shaking.

Body Temperature. Human beings and all warm-blooded animals keep an almost constant body temperature, the average daily variation being about 1° F. The normal temperature of the human body is between 96° and 99° F., the average being 98·4° F. Transient rises due to excessive heat production in vigorous exercise or to excessive external heat are soon readjusted.

Heat is produced mainly as a result of muscular and metabolic activity.

Heat is lost chiefly through the skin by the evaporation of sweat, by radiation and conduction from the surface of the body and also through the expired air from the lungs and through the excreta.

The balance of heat production and heat loss is maintained by a heat-regulating centre in the mid-brain, which is sensitive to small changes in the temperature of the circulating blood; a rise in blood temperature results in an increased flow of blood to the surface of the body, increased activity of the sweat glands with increased heat loss by evaporation. At the same time muscle tone is diminished and there is disinclination for further exercise.

A fall in the temperature of the circulating blood produces the opposite effects—constriction of the superficial blood vessels, decreased output from the sweat glands, increased muscle tone with a desire for exercise. The voluntary muscles may show the condition of reflex contraction known as shivering in an endeavour to increase heat production.

Infants and the aged are unable to adjust rapidly to changes in temperature, and are therefore more likely than the normal adult to be readily chilled by exposure to cold and more exhausted by excessive heat.

Increase in Body Temperature. A slight daily variation is shown by the normal person, the temperature being highest in the evening as the result of the day's activities, and lowest in the early morning following a night's rest.

In bacterial infections the temperature rises as a result of the increased metabolism; in diseases of the thyroid gland with over-secretion the temperature tends to be higher than normal for the same reason.

A rise of temperature above 105° F. is known as hyperpyrexia and is dangerous to the life of the body cells. Above 110° F. life cannot be long maintained.

Hyperpyrexia is found in cases of heat stroke, malaria, disorders of the central nervous system and occasionally as a complication after the operation of thyroidectomy. The temperature may be reduced by tepid sponging, evaporation of moisture and cooling of the surface of the body is greatly aided by keeping the air moving with an electric fan.

A **rigor** is a sudden disturbance of the heat regulating mechanism and commonly ushers in an acute infection— *e.g.* malaria, pneumonia, pyæmic infections. Heat production is in excess of heat loss and the temperature rapidly rises, extreme vasoconstriction makes the surface of the body feel chilly, and the patient shivers violently. This stage is followed by a stage of sudden vasodilatation, when the patient feels hot and sweats profusely, and as a result the temperature falls.

Continuous fever. The temperature rises and remains high for a period with very little fluctuation.

In typhoid fever the onset of the fever is gradual, but during the second and third week the chart shows the continuous type of fever. During the fourth week in a favourable case the temperature slowly returns to normal, such a slow defervescence being known as a fall by lysis. The course of the fever in this disease will, however, be considerably modified if the infection is cut short by successful chemotherapeutic treatment.

In lobar pneumonia unmodified by chemotherapy the temperature rises abruptly, remains high for about seven days; the fever then terminates by crisis.

Remittent Fever. In this type there are marked remissions, the evening temperature being considerably higher than the morning. This is the swinging fever seen in septic infections such as empyema and advanced tuberculosis. Occasionally the "inverse" type will be seen, when the temperature is highest in the morning and lowest in the evening.

Intermittent Fever. In this variety periods of normal temperature intermit with chills and fever. This is characteristic of malaria and may also be seen in pyæmia.

Crisis is the term used for a sudden drop from high temperature to normal within a few hours. During this time heat loss is in excess of heat production. The crisis is often accompanied by profuse sweating and polyuria and sometimes by collapse.

Post-operative Variations in Temperature. A careful

record of temperature, pulse and respiration, especially in abdominal cases, can be a valuable guide to the patient's condition and may enable the surgeon to recognize a possible complication at the earliest possible moment. A slight rise of temperature in the first twenty-four hours is usually due to reaction and not important if the pulse rate and blood pressure are normal. A low temperature with a rapid pulse indicates either a severe degree of shock or hæmorrhage.

A rise of temperature after twenty-four hours, with a slight rise in the pulse rate and a disproportionate rise of the respiratory rate, suggests chest complications. An evening rise of temperature with a corresponding rise of pulse rate from about the third day suggests sepsis.

A slight rise of temperature (about 1° F.) occurring after the seventh day may be a sign of femoral thrombosis.

Decrease in Body Temperature. A temperature below 95° is harmful to the body cells, and below 90° F. life cannot be maintained for long.

A lowering of the body temperature may be due to:

(1) Prolonged exposure to cold, especially if accompanied by starvation.

(2) Loss of fluid by hæmorrhage, excessive sweating, vomiting or diarrhœa.

(3) The condition of circulatory depression known as "shock" following severe injuries or operations.

(4) Decreased metabolic rate, *e.g.* myxœdema.

(5) Deliberate cooling of the body to a temperature 86° to 80° F. (hypothermia) for a short period in operations on the heart and great blood vessels.

An acute infection accompanied by a low or subnormal temperature and a rapid feeble pulse is a very grave condition; a sharp rise of temperature with no disproportionate rise in the pulse rate usually indicates a good reaction on the part of the body to the bacterial invasion.

In any illness a sudden fall of temperature without a general improvement in the patient's condition, and without a corresponding fall in pulse rate, is a serious sign.

To take the Temperature. The clinical thermometer is usually kept in a disinfectant, such as 1–80 phenol or in glycothymol solution, and it should be wiped free of this before use. It is very desirable that individual thermometers and containers should be provided for each patient.

The mercury must be shaken down below the lowest mark by a flick of the wrist. The thermometer should be held well in front of the nurse while doing this, to prevent accidental breakage against the bed or furniture.

The temperature may be taken in the mouth, in the rectum, or in the axilla.

The thermometer must be read immediately after it is removed, and the reading recorded before shaking down the mercury.

Taking the Temperature in the Mouth. The patient is instructed to hold the thermometer under the tongue, closing the lips, but not the teeth.

The temperature must not be taken in the mouth if the patient cannot for any reason close his mouth, if breathing is rapid or difficult, if the mouth is inflamed or sore, or if the patient is irresponsible—*e.g.* an infant, a young child, a delirious, comatose or hysterical patient.

After taking the temperature the thermometer should be washed and replaced in the container.

Taking the Temperature in the Axilla. The skin of the axilla must be dried first. The skin surfaces must meet over the thermometer, therefore, this method is not suitable in very thin patients.

The thermometer in this position will register $\frac{1}{2}°$ F. lower than in the mouth.

Taking the Temperature in the Rectum. A thermometer of special design with a thick bulb may be used. In any case thermometers used for taking rectal temperature should be kept separate from those used for taking mouth temperatures.

The thermometer should be lubricated and passed $1\frac{1}{2}$ inches into the rectum; if necessary it should be held in position. The rectal temperature is usually $\frac{1}{2}°$ to $1°$ F. higher than the mouth temperature. It gives the most reliable reading, unless the rectum is full of fæces.

Precautions. Thermometers may be marked with the time they take to register, but a minimum time of three minutes should be allowed for accurate recording.

The patient should be under the nurse's observation during the whole of this time.

Respiration

The interchange of gases between the air and the circulating blood in the air sacs of the lungs constitutes respiration. The reason for this respiratory act is the constant demand of the living cells for oxygen. The mechanism of respiration depends on the enlargement of the thoracic cavity by contractions of the intercostal muscles and the diaphragm thereby causing air to enter and expand the lungs and by the recoil of the elastic lungs, forcing air out when the chest wall relaxes. Although these muscles are voluntary muscles normal breathing is an automatic action, controlled by a centre in the medulla of the brain sensitive to the amount of carbonic acid in the blood. It is not possible to hold the breath for more than a limited time. A rise of the blood carbonic acid stimulates the centre to send urgent messages to the respiratory muscles, resulting in their contraction. Inhalation of carbonic acid gas (carbon dioxide) has the same effect, and may be an efficient method of treatment in some types of respiratory failure.

The pressure in the lungs equals atmospheric pressure, but varies a little with inspiration and expiration. The pressure in the pleural space is always negative and if, by accident or design, air is introduced into this space, equalizing the pressure there with that of the atmosphere, the lung will collapse.

All types of physical exertion increase oxygen consumption, therefore if a patient is suffering from any condition which reduces the oxygen supply to the tissues, as for example cardiac failure, complete bed rest forms an important part of his nursing care.

Taking the Respiratory Rate. The normal adult rate is between 15 and 20 per minute, but this will be increased during exercise or as a result of emotion. In infancy and childhood respiration is quicker than in the adult, being 35 to 40 in a new-born infant and about 25 per minute in a child of five years. The rate should be counted without the patient's knowledge, as control of the chest movements may be voluntary for a period. The usual method is to observe the rise and fall of the chest while still keeping the fingers on the pulse. The number of respirations may be counted for half a minute and doubled, but if there is any irregularity the count should be made for the full minute. The regularity, depth and character of the respirations should be noted at the same time.

Terms used to describe Particular Types of Respiration.

(1) *Sighing Respiration.* This is known as air hunger. Long deep inspirations, indicating a need for more oxygen, occur in cases of severe hæmorrhage and may also occur in diabetic coma, due to increased stimulation of the respiratory centre by the excess of acid in the blood.

(2) *Slow Respiration.* This is present in cases of coma due to cerebral causes or to large doses of sedative drugs. Excessively slow breathing is a characteristic of poisoning by opium or one of its derivatives.

(3) *Shallow Breathing.* This type of breathing is seen in diseases of the lung, such as pneumonia and pleurisy, when it is also rapid. Shallow breathing, which is at the same time slow, is seen in the condition of shock.

A tendency to shallow breathing is common in patients who have undergone an upper abdominal operation such as cholecystectomy or gastrectomy and deep breathing exercises are usually given in these cases.

(4) *Stertorous Breathing.* Noisy snoring inspirations occur in deeply unconscious patients and may be due to the tongue slipping back and blocking the airway. A peculiar hissing respiration may be noted in patients in uræmic coma.

(5) *Stridor.* Noisy inspiration or stridor occurs in obstruction of the upper air passages. The noise may be harsh and grating, or may be a whistling sound.

(6) *Wheezing* is the term which describes the sounds made during expiration when there is obstruction in the lower air passages, *e.g.* in cases of asthma.

(7) *Apnœa.* This term is used to denote cessation of respiration for a period.

(8) *Hyperpnœa.* Hyperpnœa means forced breathing in which the respirations are deep and rapid.

(9) *Dyspnœa.* Breathing is laboured and difficult. The difficulty may be in inspiration as in laryngeal obstruction, or in expiration as in asthma.

(10) *Orthopnœa.* This term describes the condition in which the patient is unable to breathe easily unless he is

sitting in an upright position and is frequently seen in cases of congestive cardiac failure.

(11) *Cheyne-Stokes Respiration*. This is also known as periodic breathing. It is observed in normal individuals at very high altitudes and also in patients suffering from diseases affecting the circulation of the blood and the nutrition of the respiratory centre, heart disease, renal disease, cerebral conditions and in moribund patients.

An apnœic pause is followed by shallow respirations, which gradually increase in rate and depth until, reaching a maximum, they decrease again towards another period of apnœa; the whole cycle is then repeated. After several cycles the breathing may become normal again. Since it is a serious sign, it is important to note and report this phenomenon.

Asphyxia is the name given to the condition in which the normal exchange of gases between the atmospheric air and the body tissues is interrupted. It may be due to the fact that the lungs fill with water instead of air, as in drowning, or that poisonous gases are taken up by the blood instead of oxygen—*e.g.* coal gas. It also occurs where there is obstruction of the air passages, depression of the respiratory centre, paralysis of the respiratory muscles or when the tissues are unable to take up the oxygen from the blood, as in cyanide poisoning.

For the treatment of asphyxia see pages 333–337.

The Pulse

The pulse is the wave of expansion felt in the elastic arteries when the heart pumps blood into vessels that, though always full, are distensible. The wave begins at the root of the aorta, gradually lessening as it spreads through the arterial system. In the capillaries there is normally no pulsation.

The pulse can conveniently be felt wherever a superficial artery runs over a bone—*e.g.* the radial, facial, temporal, posterior tibial and dorsalis pedis arteries.

The estimation of the rate should be made with the patient at rest. If he is not in bed, he should sit with the arm supported.

The artery is best felt by placing the index and second fingers over it. The nurse should accustom herself to the "feel" of the pulse before beginning to count the rate. An estimation of the force and rhythm of the beat should be made at the same time. Some idea may be gained also of the condition of the arterial walls.

The Pulse Rate. The frequency of the heart beat is very constant in healthy persons in the resting state, but considerable individual variation may be found. It is usually said that the average rate in the adults is 72 per minute, but rates between 50 and 90 can be regarded as within the limits of the normal. It should be borne in mind, however, that for an individual who has a normal resting pulse rate of 60, a rate of 80 to 90 would be abnormal. In infancy the pulse rate is 120 to 140, at the age of three years about 100. In old age the rate tends to slow down.

Physiological Variations in the Normal Individual. Active muscular exercise may double the resting pulse rate, but there is quick return to normal after a short rest. Emotion also quickens the heart beat. These physiological increases enable the heart to increase its output per minute and so increase the blood supply to the working muscle. In the trained athlete, however, the heart responds to exercise with an increased strength of the beat without any great increase in rate.

The heart beats more slowly in any condition in which the metabolic rate is decreased—*e.g.* complete rest, starvation.

Pathological Alterations in the Pulse Rate

Tachycardia is the term used to denote a quick action of the heart. The commonest conditions in which the rate is increased are:

(1) Fever, with the accompanying increased metabolic rate. The pulse rate usually rises 10 beats per minute for every 1° F. rise of temperature above 99°.

(2) Increased activity of the thyroid gland (thyrotoxicosis).

(3) Lessened oxygen-carrying capacity of the blood in hæmorrhage and anæmia.

(4) Nervous disorders of the heart beat, paroxysmal tachycardia.

(5) A failing heart muscle; in any severe illness a rapid pulse which is also feeble is a very grave sign.

(6) Auricular fibrillation uncontrolled by digitalis.

(7) The action of drugs—*e.g.* atropine, amyl nitrite.

Bradycardia means a slow action of the heart. This is found in:

(1) Stimulation of the vagus control of the heart by drugs or by increased intracranial pressure, such as may occur in cerebral tumour, cerebral injuries or hæmorrhage.

(2) Narcotic drugs—*e.g.* opium.

(3) Decreased activity of the thyroid gland (myxœdema).

(4) A slow pulse may be found in neurasthenic conditions and in convalescence after serious illness.

(5) Disease of the conducting tissue of the heart—"heart block." In heart block the pulse may be between 30 and 40. Digitalis slows the heart through its effect on the conducting tissue.

(6) A slow pulse is often noted in cases of jaundice.

Rhythm. Where any irregularity in rhythm is noted the pulse should be counted for a complete minute; if it is counted only for a quarter of a minute there is a greater opportunity for error. In such cases the apex beat of the heart should also be counted with the stethoscope, and both rates should be charted.

An entirely irregular pulse will show variations both in rhythm and strength. Some irregularities are not important, but when noted should always be reported.

Sinus Arrhythmia. This is a condition in which the pulse quickens on inspiration and slows on expiration. It may be noticed in children and young people and is of no significance.

Extra Systole. This is an intermittent pulse. An extra beat is followed by an abnormally long pause, the patient may be conscious of this and may say that the "heart stops." In young people it may be due to irritation from excessive smoking, fatigue, or a septic focus; in the older patient it is more likely to indicate some degeneration of the heart muscle.

A completely irregular pulse is found in *auricular fibrillation*. The auricles contract very rapidly and very feebly; the rate may be 200 to 300 per minute. These feeble contractions are not all transmitted to the ventricles, but although the ventricular rate is slower than the auricular rate, the ventricles are also beating quickly and irregularly. Some of the ventricular contractions occur when the ventricle is incompletely filled and the pulse wave may not be felt at the wrist (pulse deficit). It is therefore necessary to record both the pulse rate and the heart apex beat as heard with a stethoscope.

Digitalis is more often ordered in auricular fibrillation than any other drug and may cause slowing of the heart rate and the abnormality known as "coupling," in which two beats of unequal force are followed by an extra long pause. The nurse should keep a careful watch on the pulse. Coupling is often the first symptom of overdose of digitalis.

Blood Pressure

Blood pressure is the force which the circulating blood exerts upon its enclosing walls, and is maintained by:

(1) The force of the heart beat.

(2) The tone of the vessel walls.

(3) The amount of fluid in circulation.

(4) The viscosity of the fluid.

The blood pressure must be maintained at a certain level to keep up the supply to the heart muscle and the vital centres in the brain. The average force of the pressure in the large arteries when the heart is actively pumping is sufficient to support a column of mercury 120 mm. high, therefore the average systolic pressure is said to be 120. The pressure when the heart is resting is about two-thirds of the systolic pressure, this is the diastolic pressure. The difference between the systolic and diastolic pressure gives the pulse pressure—*e.g.* if the systolic pressure is 120 mm. of mercury and the diastolic pressure is 80 mm., then the pulse pressure is 40 mm. The average range of the systolic pressure in an adult—between 30 and 40 years old—is 110 to 140 mm.

In women the average pressure is 5 to 10 mm. lower than in men.

At birth the average systolic pressure is 30 to 40 mm.

Other factors which affect the blood pressure are:

(1) Exercise and emotional excitement, which raise the pressure.

(2) Change of position. The pressure is lower in the recumbent than in the erect position.

A rise in pressure may be due to:

(1) Loss of elasticity of the vessel walls. Hardened arteries offer a greater resistance to the circulating blood and

therefore the pressure rises. The condition commonly referred to as apoplexy or a stroke may result from rupture of vessels in the brain. Congestive heart failure may also result from the persistent extra burden on the heart.

(2) Fever. With a raised temperature and increased metabolism the pressure commonly rises, but with severe infection and marked toxæmia (*e.g.* diphtheria) the pressure may fall.

(3) In chronic renal disease the pressure rises and a high blood pressure may be present before renal efficiency tests or the presence of albumen show diminished kidney function.

A sustained rise in blood pressure is known as *hypertension*; in many cases no cause can be found for this.

A fall in pressure may be due to:

(1) Surgical shock.

(2) Any sudden catastrophe, such as a coronary thrombosis.

(3) Excessive loss of fluid from hæmorrhage, diarrhœa or vomiting.

(4) Disease of the suprarenal glands, with deficient secretion (Addison's disease).

(5) Debility in convalescence and lack of tone in the vascular system.

Serious and sudden falls in the blood pressure are treated by keeping the head low and raising the lower part of the trunk and the legs, by the administration of fluids to increase the blood volume, and by drugs which will constrict the vessel walls and so raise the pressure (*e.g.* adrenaline and pituitrin). In severe hæmorrhage the fall in pressure by reducing the force of the circulation tends to check the bleeding, therefore the bleeding should be controlled before active measures are taken to raise the blood pressure.

A persistently low blood pressure is known as *hypotension*.

Estimation of the Blood Pressure. The pressure is recorded in millimetres of mercury by an apparatus known as the sphygmomanometer. The usual type has a mercury gauge connected with the rubber cuff which can be inflated by a hand pump. The cuff is fixed evenly round the arm above the elbow with the centre over the brachial artery. The arm should be resting on the bed or on a table.

The pressure in the cuff is raised by pumping until it is

sufficient to obliterate the radial artery. The pressure is
then very gradually reduced by letting air escape until the
pulse becomes just perceptible. The height of the mercury
column at this point is the systolic pressure. The apparatus
should be placed so that the patient cannot see the mercury
column. The procedure should be first explained to the
patient so that he understands that it is not a painful one.

**The Auscultatory Method of estimating Systolic and
Diastolic Pressure.** A sphygmomanometer and a stethoscope are needed. This method requires considerable
practice.

The patient sits or lies with the arm supported and the
sphygmomanometer cuff applied. Absolute silence is
essential. Before inflating the cuff the brachial artery must
be located on the inner side of the biceps muscle. The
pressure in the armlet is raised until the radial pulse is
obliterated. The stethoscope is applied over the brachial
artery and the pressure is very gradually reduced.

When the pressure falls to the systolic level a series of
tapping sounds is heard as the blood begins to flow through
the artery. The pressure at which the first of these taps is
heard is the systolic level. With the pressure reduced a
little lower the tapping sounds are replaced by a soft murmur,
still lower by a series of loud clear sounds like the beats of
a gong. With a slight further reduction in pressure these
sounds change to a dull muffled note which is heard during
the next 5–6 mm. of fall, after which no further sounds are
heard. The level of the mercury as the muffled sounds
disappear is the reading of the diastolic pressure.

Charting

Making a chart is a graphic way of recording various data
so that variations are readily appreciated by the eye.

It is the method by which variations in the temperature
are most easily recorded, and the value of the chart is greatly
increased if the pulse and respiratory rates and the blood
pressure are also charted in the same way.

Where there is no reason to expect any sudden change
in any of these signs a morning and evening chart is used.
If there is fever, the temperature, pulse and respiration are
recorded four-hourly. In certain cases hourly or half-hourly
charts of the pulse and/or blood pressure readings are kept.

A chart should be neatly and accurately kept and it is best to use a fine pen. Any written details should be in small but legible writing. The record of temperature, pulse and respiration, with notes on the action of the bowels, the quantity of urine passed, the amount of vomit or sputum, if any, are usually kept in a book and charted daily. Records of the patient's fluid intake and fluid output are in many cases of great importance and the amounts are usually entered on a special form. The records should be made immediately whenever fluid is given and whenever fluid is lost by passing urine or by other routes, as for example by vomiting. The figures should be written in ordinary Arabic numerals, the use of Roman numerals may be a source of error, *e.g.* IX when written hurriedly may look very like IV, and in any case they are less quickly written and less easily read than the Arabic figures. Where a four-hourly chart is used the temperature, pulse and respiration should be charted as soon as taken. All special treatments and drugs are usually entered on the chart when given.

The aim in keeping a chart is to give as much information as possible regarding the patient's condition and treatment. The only permissible gaps in the temperature, pulse and respiration records are when the patient is sleeping and disturbance would be detrimental to his progress.

8

Feeding Sick People: Infant Feeding: Invalid Cookery

FEEDING sick people is a very important part of medical treatment and of nursing care alike. Recently a great deal of attention has been centred on the application of the science of nutrition to the preservation of health and the prevention of disease.

The requirements of a satisfactory diet are a sufficient amount of the body-building and fuel foods, water and accessory or regulatory substances, the vitamins and mineral salts.

A certain amount of indigestible material should form a part of the daily diet of the normal person to promote peristalsis and elimination.

The fuel value of the diet is calculated in terms of calories, and the energy value required will vary according to the age, occupation and environment of the individual, but it is commonly taken to be between 2,500 and 3,000 calories per day. A calorie is the amount of heat required to raise the temperature of 1 kilogramme of water 1° C.

The energy-giving foods are the proteins, carbohydrates and fats.

Protein. Protein is used for tissue building as well as for fuel, and is obtained from meat, fish, eggs, milk and milk products; also to some extent from vegetable sources, wheat, rye, peas, beans and nuts. When burnt as fuel, proteins yield 4 calories per gramme. The protein requirement is about 1 gramme for every kilogramme of body weight, or about 15 per cent. of the total daily requirements.

Carbohydrates. These have the same energy-giving value as proteins; they are cheaper and represent about 50 to 60 per cent. of the daily diet. The chief sources are cereals, potatoes, root vegetables, sugars and fruits.

Fats. When burnt in the body, fat gives more than double the energy value of starches and sugars (9 calories per gramme), but are more difficult to digest and metabolize. Fats are also required for certain of the body tissues such as the nerve sheaths and cell envelopes, for the cholesterol in the bile and the secretion of the sebaceous glands. Fat is the chief form in which the body stores fuel.

Fats are comparatively costly sources of energy and form approximately 30 per cent. of an average diet.

It should be remembered that, as commonly eaten, most foods contain a certain proportion of waste and very few are pure sources of any one substance. Sugar may be mentioned as a pure carbohydrate, butter is almost pure fat, but contains a varying amount of water.

Water. Water is essential to life, and a fair proportion is taken into the body with the various foods; in addition, about 3 pints in the twenty-four hours should be drunk. This is, of course, not all taken as plain water, but as the various beverages in common use, *e.g.* tea, coffee, lemonade and fruit juices.

The Vitamins. These are factors essential for maintaining normal health and metabolism. They are not likely to be deficient in a good mixed diet, but especial care is needed in restricted diets to ensure that they are present in adequate amounts.

The vitamins A, D, E and K are classed as the fat-soluble vitamins. A is essential for the growth of young animals and also is considered to play some part as an "anti-infective" agent. Good sources are butter, cream, egg yolk, fish oils, carrots and green vegetables. Vegetable oils are deficient in vitamin A, therefore vitamin A and also vitamin D are added to margarine.

Vitamin D controls the use of calcium and phosphorus in the body and is called the antirachitic factor. It is more stable to heat than A. Good sources are cod- and halibut-liver oils, egg yolk and butter. Vitamin D is built up in the deeper layers of the skin when a sterol present in the skin is irradiated with ultra-violet light, therefore, sunshine will prevent and to a certain extent cure rickets, however deficient the diet may be in vitamin D. Pure vitamin D is known as calciferol.

Vitamin E is known as the antisterility factor: experiments

have suggested that a deficiency of this vitamin causes sterility in rats, but there is little evidence of its effect on human beings. Good sources are green leaves, whole grains, egg yolk and fresh meat.

Vitamin K, the antihæmorrhagic factor, is necessary for the normal clotting of blood. Natural sources of this vitamin are cabbage, spinach and fruits. A chemical substance Kapilon almost identical with vitamin K can be given by hypodermic injection.

Vitamins B and C are water-soluble.

The vitamin B complex is a series of vitamins all found in considerable amounts in yeast and the germ of cereals. B_1 is necessary for the regulation of carbohydrate metabolism. In addition to yeast and the germ of cereals, this vitamin is also present in egg yolk, fresh vegetables and fruit. Vitamin B_1 in the pure state is known as aneurine. Nicotinic acid, or the pellagra-preventing factor, is also a part of the vitamin B complex; yeast, cereals, eggs, milk and liver are all good sources. Riboflavine (vitamin B_2) is thought to be responsible in part for oxidative changes in the tissue cells. Some of the symptoms of pellagra are due to deficiency of this factor. Riboflavine is found in milk, liver and yeast. Vitamin B_{12}, or cyanocobalamin, is found in liver and is a part of the anti-anæmic factor.

Vitamin C prevents scurvy. It is easily destroyed at high temperatures, especially in conjunction with alkalis such as soda. Good sources are raw green vegetables, swedes, tomatoes and the citrous fruits, especially oranges. Pure vitamin C is known as ascorbic acid.

The Mineral Salts. These are especially important during the early period of life, although a good supply of calcium is necessary also in the diet of the pregnant woman in order to supply material for the bones and teeth of the developing fœtus. The chief inorganic substances required are sodium, calcium, phosphorus and iron. Iodine in very small amounts is needed for the secretion of the thyroid gland. A good mixed diet of animal and vegetable foods gives an ample supply of these substances. Milk and cheese are particularly rich sources of calcium, but are deficient in iron. Meat and green vegetables are a good source of iron.

In disease the diet may be restricted, the balance or the

texture of the diet may be altered, the calorie value may be increased or decreased. For information on the science of nutrition and the dietetic treatment of disease the student should consult a textbook of dietetics.

Hospital Diets

Patients' diets (with the exception of those ordered for patients suffering from diseases in which special feeding is an important part of the treatment of the disease) served in hospital wards are commonly classed as "full," "light" and "fluid." In the past, dietary scales showing the amount of such foods as meat, fish, milk, eggs, butter and sugar which could be ordered for patients on the various grades of diet were commonly used. However, partly as a result of the attention which war-time rationing directed upon the provision of an adequate, if restricted, diet, and partly as a result of greater knowledge of nutrition, the feeding of patients and staff in hospitals has been under review and the importance of the catering departments of such establishments has been rightly emphasized. Most hospitals have a catering committee which considers all aspects of the subject, buying supplies, planning the dietary, cooking and serving meals. The successful operation of many very large canteens for industrial workers has shown that the problems of good service of well cooked meals can be solved. A very interesting memorandum on hospital diet prepared by King Edward Hospital Fund for London states that "the food service should be regarded as one of the essential remedial services offered by the hospitals." The memorandum also adds that hospitals have an opportunity of educating the public in sound principles of feeding.

Serving Meals

The nurse's part in the food service of the hospital is an important one as she is the person who presents it to the patient. It is essential that hot meals should be conveyed to the ward and served with the minimum of delay. All trays should be set beforehand, the kitchen prepared for this service and hot plates ready. Every nurse should consider it her responsibility to see that the best use is made of the food sent to the ward. If some simple cookery, such as boiling eggs for patients' breakfasts, is expected of her

5+

she should take a pride in doing this well. The art of cutting thin bread and butter and attractive sandwiches is well worth acquiring. Quite apart from the question of the patient's enjoyment of his meal it is obvious that poor cooking and indifferent service will result in considerable food wastage.

Food which looks tempting stimulates both the salivary and gastric secretion, so that digestion is aided. A badly served meal arouses a feeling of disgust, and the digestive functions are inhibited instead of helped.

Absolute cleanliness of the tray itself, the tray cloth and all utensils is essential. Glass and cutlery should be clean and shining.

All condiments allowed should be ready on the tray. The patient's appetite should be taken into consideration; if it is small, only small portions should be served at first and a second helping offered. Only one course is served at a time. The tray should contain nothing that the patient is forbidden, and should not be crowded with unnecessary articles. If the patient can feed himself, he should be settled in a comfortable position and the tray placed where he can conveniently reach it.

Hot food must be really hot; hot drinks should be at the right temperature and not boiling. Cold food should be served cold and not tepid. Special feeds must be served punctually at the time ordered. Any complaints made by patients should at once be reported to the sister, and she should also be told if any patients have not eaten what was served.

Trays should be cleared away promptly and the crockery and cutlery neatly stacked in the kitchen ready for the ward maid.

Feeding Helpless Patients

If a helpless patient has to be fed with a full diet he should be allowed time to eat properly, and not made to feel that the nurse is anxious for him to finish as quickly as possible. The patient should be supported in a comfortable position and the nurse should be seated at the right hand side of the bed facing the patient.

A helpless patient on a fluid diet is usually fed with a spouted feeder. The patient is told that he can control the flow of the liquid by putting his tongue over the opening of the spout; the feeder should be tilted sufficiently to allow him to get a good drink. If he is very weak, then he must be fed with small sips, and a spoon may be better than a feeding cup. The best method of supporting the patient's head while he drinks is to put an arm under his pillow raising this and the patient's head together.

Children who have not been trained to eat properly may require a great deal of kind, but firm, supervision at meal times. The nurse cannot deal too firmly with a sick child who has developed many likes and dislikes over his food, but during a long stay in hospital the nurses can do a great deal to instil good habits into the child. If he can feed himself, it is usually better to let him do so, but his gown should be protected by a bib and the sheet by a cloth. Children as a rule demand frequent drinks of water, and in most cases this want should be satisfied. Sweets and fruit are best given after meals, and extra articles of food brought in should be given into the charge of the ward sister.

Infant Feeding

During the early months of life the natural food of the infant is breast milk.

The first secretion from the mammary glands is colostrum. This first food is nature's way of accustoming the infant stomach to the presence of food and starting the action of sucking. It contains some protein and protective bodies against certain infections.

On the third day after delivery the mammary glands secrete milk. This food is supplied at the correct temperature and its composition is suited to the needs of the infant. The bacterial content is very low. In some cases the breast milk may be insufficient, but, if possible, every infant should be breast fed for at least the first few months of life, unless there is any obvious contra-indication such as active tuberculosis in the mother.

The mother's diet must contain the necessary raw materials for the manufacture of good milk and she often needs to be told of the necessity for drinking plenty of water.

Artificial feeding may be used to supplement or to replace breast feeding. The majority of sick infants in hospital are artificially fed. If, however, breast feeding is continued, the mother must attend at the stated times and provision made for her privacy and comfort.

The actual feeds ordered will, of course, vary with the age and condition of the infant.

Cow's milk used for infant feeding should come from a reliable dairy and, unless from tuberculin-tested cows, the milk must be either boiled or pasteurized. Dried milk powder is, however, more frequently used than fresh milk. The protein and fat are more finely divided than in fresh milk, and so may be more easily digested by the sick baby. Recipes for the preparation of special feeds such as lactic acid milk, butter-flour mixture and thickened feeds will be found at the end of the chapter.

All utensils used for mixing and preparing feeds must be kept solely for that purpose, and the prepared feeds are best kept in an ice chest or refrigerator.

Accuracy in measurements and scrupulous cleanliness are essential in the preparation of the feeds.

It is common practice to give orange juice and cod- or halibut-liver oil daily to ensure the presence of the necessary A, C and D vitamins, as the vitamin content of milk is very variable.

The bottle used for artificial feeding may be either a straight one with a rubber teat at the end or the boat-shaped bottle with a valve at one end and a teat at the other. The hole in the rubber teat should be sufficiently large to allow the fluid to drop through, but not big enough to allow the infant to take the feed too quickly. If the infant can be taken from his cot at feeding time, he should be supported on the nurse's left arm in an almost sitting position. An interval should be allowed half-way through, and the time taken for the whole feed should be between ten and fifteen minutes.

After use the bottle should be washed with cold water, then with warm soapy water, rinsed well and boiled. It may be kept in a covered sterile bowl when not in use.

Teats are cleaned by first washing well on both sides, using a soft brush. Salt is rubbed over the inside and outside and the teat is then well rinsed in cold water boiled, and stored in a small covered jar or cup.

From the age of four months or earlier, additions are made gradually to the diet. The first additions are usually cereals, meat gravy and sieved vegetables, later grated cheese, eggs, potato, milk puddings and fruit pulp may be given.

Sick-Room Cookery

Cooking food increases its digestibility and improves and develops the flavour, thereby stimulating appetite; it destroys bacteria and parasites, and delays the putrefactive processes.

Food for invalids should be fresh and of the best quality obtainable. Variety should as far as possible be introduced, and the individual likes and dislikes of patients studied. It should be cooked in the simplest and most digestible ways, these are steaming, boiling, grilling or baking. As a general rule highly seasoned dishes and fried food are unsuitable. Meat, fish and eggs should not be overcooked, as the protein becomes hard and difficult to digest. Starchy foods are rendered more easily digestible by prolonged cooking.

BARLEY WATER (1)

Ingredients: 2 tablespoonfuls of pearl barley.
1 lemon.
2 tablespoonfuls of sugar.
2 pints water.

Method. Wash the barley and put in the saucepan with the thinly peeled rind of the lemon. Simmer gently for one and a half to two hours. Strain and add the lemon juice and sugar. Grape fruit may be used instead of lemon.

BARLEY WATER (2)

A quick method may be used which makes a thinner drink preferred by many patients.

Method. The barley and lemon rind are placed in a warm jug and one pint of boiling water is added. The jug is covered and left to cool. Lemon juice and sugar are added to taste.

IMPERIAL DRINK

Ingredients: 1 teaspoonful of cream of tartar.
3 to 4 oz. sugar.
Juice of 1 lemon.
1 pint boiling water.

Method. Put the cream of tartar, sugar and lemon juice

in a jug. Pour on the boiling water and stir well. Cover and use cold, diluting with plain water, barley water or soda water.

SIMPLE DILUTION OF COW'S MILK FOR INFANT FEEDING

Ingredients: 10 oz. milk.
10 oz. water.
1 oz. lactose, or sugar.
1 oz. double cream (48 per cent. fat).

Cod-liver oil may replace some of the cream. Roughly the composition is: Protein, 2 per cent.; fat, 4 per cent.; carbohydrate, 6 per cent. Calorie value, 20 calories to the ounce.

N.B. Dried milk is more often used than fresh cow's milk.

BUTTER-FLOUR MIXTURE

Ingredients: 3 level tablespoonfuls of butter.
5 level tablespoonfuls of wheat flour.
2 level tablespoonfuls of sugar.
20 oz. water.
Milk to make up 1 quart.

Method. Cook the butter for five minutes in a saucepan. Add the wheat flour and cook together for a further five minutes, stirring continuously to prevent the mixture from getting lumpy. Add the sugar and the pint of water, cooking again for twenty minutes. Milk is then added to make the whole mixture up to 1 quart.

Composition: Fat, 5·8 per cent.; carbohydrate, 9 per cent.; protein, 2·2 per cent. Calorie value, 30 calories per ounce.

THICKENED MILK FEED

Ingredients: 6 tablespoonfuls of flour.
20 oz. milk.

Method. Mix the flour to a smooth paste with sufficient cold milk. Add the remainder of the pint of milk slowly. Cook the mixture in a double saucepan until the volume is reduced to 15 oz. and the mixture is of a jelly consistency.

Composition: Fat, 4·8 per cent.; protein, 5·5 per cent.; carbohydrate, 16 per cent. Calorie value, 40 calories per ounce.

Lactic Acid Milk

Ingredients: 60 minims lactic acid, B.P.
1 pint milk.

Method. The acid is added drop by drop, stirring all the time, as if making mayonnaise. A very fine curd is formed. Cane sugar, honey or dextrimaltose may be added. Without the addition of sugar, the composition and caloric value will be the same as cow's milk.

Milk Vegetable Soup

Ingredients: ½ pint milk.
Small piece of carrot, onion, celery and lettuce (if available) and turnip.
½ oz. butter.
½ oz. flour, lightly seasoned.
2 tablespoonfuls of cream if desired.

Method. Peel turnip, scrape carrot, skin onion, cut vegetables into fine shreds, sauté them in the butter in a saucepan (do not let them take colour), sprinkle in seasoned flour and cook. Add milk gradually, and bring to simmering point. Cook about twenty minutes, or until vegetables are tender. Serve very hot, with toast.

Baked Custard

Ingredients: 1 egg.
½ pint milk.
1 dessertspoonful of sugar.

Method. Grease the pie dish. Beat the egg and add the sugar and milk warmed, and pour into the pie dish. Place in a tin of cold water in the middle of a warm oven and allow to cook slowly, raising to the top shelf to brown.

Egg Jelly

Ingredients: ½ pint of liquid made up of the strained juice of 1 lemon and water.
Peel of 1 lemon thinly cut.
2 oz. loaf sugar, or to taste.
1 egg.
¼ oz. gelatine.

Method. Put all ingredients except the egg into a lined saucepan. Beat the egg and add, beating all the time. Stir over a very low heat with a fork until the gelatine is dissolved. The mixture *must not boil or it will curdle.*

Cool, strain, mould, and when set turn out on to a small dish.

ORANGE JELLY

Ingredients: ½ pint of liquid consisting of juice of 2 oranges and 1 lemon.
¼ oz. gelatine.
Rind of 1 orange and ½ lemon thinly cut.
2 oz. of sugar.

Method. Put all the ingredients into a lined saucepan. Stir over a very gentle heat until the gelatine is dissolved. Cool, strain and mould.

BREAD AND BUTTER PUDDING

Ingredients: 1½ gills milk.
1 egg.
1 dessertspoonful of sugar.
1 tablespoonful of clean sultanas.
2 or 3 slices (thin) of bread and butter.

Method. Grease pie dish well. Beat egg and milk together. Place bread and butter in dish (butter side downwards), sprinkle sultanas over, then add another layer of bread and butter. Pour custard over; stand aside for ½ hour. Grate nutmeg over, if liked. Stand in tin of water; bake slowly until custard is set and the top a pale brown. Serve immediately.

SCRAMBLED EGGS

Ingredients: 1 or 2 new-laid eggs.
1 dessertspoonful of milk (for 2 eggs).
Piece of butter (size of walnut).
Slice of hot buttered toast.
Pepper and salt.

Method. Make toast, butter it and keep hot. Beat eggs a little with milk. Add pepper and salt. Melt butter in saucepan, pour in egg mixture, and cook slowly, stirring well until the egg is nearly set. Pile upon toast; garnish with parsley. Serve at once.

JUNKET

Ingredients: ½ pint milk.
Essence of rennet (quantity according to instructions on bottle).

1 teaspoonful of castor sugar.

Nutmeg or other flavouring, if desired.

Method. The junket bowls must be dry. Dissolve the sugar in the milk, making the milk luke-warm (temperature 98° to 100° F.). Add the rennet and pour into junket bowls. Grate the nutmeg over the milk and leave until set.

Steamed Whiting and Parsley Sauce

Method. Fillet and skin fish when necessary. Lay on board, skinned side up, season, squeeze a few drops of lemon juice over and roll up. Grease a soup plate, place the fish on the plate and cover with a greased paper and a saucepan lid. Place over a saucepan of boiling water; cook for about twenty minutes. Liquid from the fish should be used for the sauce, making up the required quanitity of fluid with milk.

Sauce

Ingredients: ½ oz. butter.
½ oz. flour.
7 oz. liquid (milk, or milk and liquid from fish).
1 teaspoonful of chopped parsley.

Method. Melt the butter in a small saucepan. Remove from the heat and stir in the flour. Return the saucepan to the gas and cook slowly for about six minutes, but do not brown. Add the liquid slowly, beating well until free from lumps. Boil for eight minutes. Add the chopped parsley. Coat the fish and serve.

High Protein Drinks

Used to increase the protein content of the diet as for example in the treatment of malnutrition, nephrosis, and liver damage.

Ingredients: 10 oz. milk.
3 oz. dried skim milk.
½ oz. soluble protein (casein).
8 oz. water.

Protein value, 55 grammes;

Calorie value, 540.

Method. Measure the milk into a china bowl and whisk in the dried skim milk and the soluble protein. Add the water and strain. The drink may be served warm or cold

5*

sweetened and flavoured according to taste with coffee, cocoa, etc. The mixture must not be boiled as this will coagulate the soluble protein.

A proprietary preparation, Complan, is a convenient and palatable high protein drink.

9

Tube Feeding (Artificial Feeding)

General Considerations

TUBE feeding is the term used to describe the administration of fluid food through a tube passed into the stomach either through the patient's mouth or nose or through an artificial opening.

Any form of tube feeding is undertaken only on the doctor's orders.

If the treatment is to be carried out for the first time, or if the patient is restive, it is necessary to have the help of a second nurse.

The feed should be given slowly at a temperature of 100° F.

Absolute cleanliness is essential in the preparation of the feed, and the tray should look as attractive as possible.

Privacy for the patient should be ensured.

Properly carried out, the procedure should not cause pain or marked discomfort.

If artificial feeding is continued for more than a few days, care must be taken in planning the diet to ensure that it is sufficient in calorie value and contains the essential accessory factors. A fluid balance chart should be accurately kept.

Frequent cleaning of the mouth must be carried out. Chewing gum will help to keep mouth and teeth in a healthy condition.

The Oral Route

This procedure, although comparatively seldom used now, may be ordered for mental patients refusing food, in cases of paralysis of the soft palate or the swallowing muscles, for unconscious patients and, in some cases, after operations on the pharynx, larynx or trachea.

Requirements:

An œsophageal catheter, size 14 to 22 (for post-

operative pharyngeal or laryngeal cases a much
smaller tube, size 8 to 12, may be required).

A glass funnel.

A piece of rubber tubing to fit the glass funnel.

A glass connection to attach the tubing to the œsophageal tube.

A measure containing sterile water at a temperature of
100° F.

A measure containing the feed standing in a bowl of
warm water.

A lotion thermometer.

A bowl for the apparatus.

A mackintosh bib and feeding cloth.

Mouth tray and mouth wash.

Squares of old linen for wiping the mouth.

A gag if the patient is unconscious or resistant.

The Feed. 10 to 15 oz. may be given at two-, four- or six-
hour intervals according to orders. Milk forms the basis,
but various other foods such as eggs beaten up, sugar, malted
milk powder or chocolate may be added to increase the
nutritive value of the feed.

Method. The patient is unlikely to be wearing dentures,
but if he should be, these must first be removed. He may
be sitting up or lying on his left side. The mouth should
be cleaned and the gag inserted if required. The tube
should be passed over the tongue, guiding the tip so that it
does not strike the posterior pharyngeal wall. If the patient
is conscious, he should be directed to swallow and then
given time to breathe before being asked to swallow again.
The tube should have marks at 16 and 18 inches from the
tip and 17 to 18 inches should be passed.

When the tube is in the stomach it should be compressed
to expel the air. The feed should be poured in slowly and
a little water poured down the tube afterwards. The tube
should then be pinched tightly and removed in one quick
movement. The mouth should be cleaned or the patient
given a mouth wash.

The Nasal Route

This is more commonly used than the oral route. It may
be used in cases of weakly infants unable to suck, unconscious
patients, after operations on the mouth, pharynx or larynx

in cases of pharyngeal paralysis or in the treatment of gastric conditions.

Requirements:

A barrel of a glass syringe or a small glass funnel.

A fine catheter, size 4 for infants, size 6 for older children; for an adult a small size œsophageal tube is used. A Ryle's duodenal tube may also be used.

A piece of rubber tubing to fit the glass barrel, about 8 inches long.

A glass connection.

Boracic lotion and ointment.

Wool swabs.

A mackintosh bib and feeding cloth.

A bowl for the apparatus.

A measure containing sterile water.

A measure containing the feed standing in a bowl of warm water.

A lotion thermometer.

If a lubricant is required, butter or liquid paraffin may be used.

The Feed. This will vary according to the age and condition of the patient. The basis of the feed is usually milk; glucose or cane sugar, protein and vitamin preparations may be added.

Method. The patient may be lying on his back or sitting up. In the case of a child an assistant will restrain movements by wrapping the child in a blanket and also help by steadying the head. The mackintosh and feeding cloth should then be arranged. One nostril should be gently cleaned with a small swab wrung out of the boracic lotion. The tube should be passed along the floor of the nose backwards and downwards.

If the patient is conscious he will cough and splutter if the tube tries to enter the larynx, in this event the tube should be withdrawn and passed again. If the patient is deeply unconscious the laryngeal reflex is lost and he will not cough, but may become cyanosed if the tube is in the air passage, this again is an indication for immediate withdrawal of the tube.

Tests should be carried out before giving the feed to make sure that the tube has passed down the œsophagus and is in the stomach. The funnel may be attached to the tube and then placed in a bowl of water, should the tube be in the air passages this will be indicated by bubbles of air. A better test is to attach a syringe to the end of the tube and to aspirate the stomach contents as proof of the position of the tube before any fluid is poured down. If there is any doubt about the position of the tube or if any difficulty is experienced in passing it, the doctor should be asked to verify that all is well before the nurse proceeds with the feeding.

The feed should be poured in slowly, holding the funnel only slightly above the level of the patient's head. When it is finished a little sterile water should be poured down the tube, which when empty is pinched tightly near the nostril and removed in one quick movement. The nostril should be cleaned and a little boracic ointment applied to prevent soreness. Alternate nostrils should be used.

If nasal feeding is required over a period of several days the tube may be left in position between the feedings. It is usual to change the tube every twenty-four hours. If continuous feeding is required the nasal tube is attached to a container with a drip connection.

Gastrostomy Feeding

When the operation of gastrostomy is performed for the purpose of feeding a patient, a catheter (usually a self-retaining one, such as a De Pezzer catheter) is put into the stomach through an incision made in the abdominal wall and the stomach wall. The tube is taken out periodically and replaced by a new one.

It is especially important in the first few days after the operation to notice if the tube slips out of the opening, as it should be replaced at once. If it remains out for any length of time it may be very difficult to replace. Should the nurse have to replace it, she should remember the danger of pushing it between the abdominal wall and the stomach wall into the peritoneal cavity. The tube should be inserted without force into the centre of the opening.

Requirements:
Glass funnel.
Piece of rubber tubing.
Tubing clip.
Glass connection.

A catheter, if the gastrostomy tube has been removed
and the opening closed by gastrostomy plug.

Mackintosh.

Clean dressing and bandage, if likely to be required.

Measure containing water.

Bowl for apparatus.

If the gastrostomy tube has not been removed and the
outer opening is closed by a spigot, a clean spigot
should be provided to close the tube after the feed
has been given.

The Feed. As the usual reason for a gastrostomy is a
malignant stricture of the œsophagus, the patient is probably
emaciated from months of starvation. It is important that
he should receive a diet which is adequate in nutritive
quality and also containing the necessary accessory constituents of a balanced diet. A diet with a calorie value of
2,500 to 3,000 is desirable. The patient if properly fed,
should regain and retain some at least of his lost weight and
strength.

Feeding is begun as soon as he recovers from the anæsthetic, and at first small quantities are given, but those are
soon increased.

Any food that will pass down the tube may be given.
Milk forms the basis, with the addition of eggs, cream,
lactose and soluble protein. Soup may be given with
Marmite added for the vitamin B value. Orange juice given
once a day keeps up the supply of vitamin C.

Method. The mackintosh is arranged to protect the
dressing.

The spigot is removed from the catheter, or if the catheter
has been removed the gastrostomy plug is taken out and
the catheter required for feeding inserted into the opening.

The end of the glass connection is fixed to the catheter
in the gastrostomy opening.

The tubing is compressed to expel air. The feed is given
slowly, finishing with water to wash through the catheter, if
this is omitted the catheter may be blocked by coagulation of the milk as a result of the action of the gastric juice.

The glass connection, tubing and funnel are removed and
the spigot or the gastrostomy plug, whichever is used, is
replaced. The gastric contents are very irritating to the
skin should they leak through the tube, therefore a protective

cream or ointment is applied to the skin around the opening.

The patient is usually taught to give his own feeds before leaving hospital.

Jejunostomy Feeding

An opening made into the jejunum may be used for feeding in a similar manner to the gastrostomy. The jejunostomy is usually made in cases where the stomach is unable to tolerate any food, as in very large ulcers or new growth of the stomach.

The jejunum can accommodate only very small amounts, so that feeding has to be carried out at very short intervals. The food may be pre-digested. The skin around the opening must be protected by an ointment or paint.

Mouth Feeding in Special Cases

Operations and injuries of the mouth preventing the patient from eating in the normal way call for special management.

(1) **Harelip.** Infants with this congenital deformity are unable to suck naturally, and are fed with a spoon or a pipette, or by nasal catheter.

For spoon feeding the infant should be laid flat on the nurse's lap and the milk put into the hollow of the cheek and well to the back of the mouth.

If the child is spoon fed after operations on the lip, a small narrow spoon should be used. It is essential not to stretch the mouth or to allow the spoon to touch the upper lip.

The infant must have sufficient nourishment, and should not be allowed to cry from hunger or for any other reason, as apart from the discomfort that the infant may suffer, crying may damage the repaired lip.

(2) **Cleft Palate.** After operation the child is usually fed through a spouted feeder with a piece of rubber tubing attached. Cold liquids are given at first, with a drink of sterile water after every feed to cleanse the mouth.

The surgeon will decide how soon the child may have food requiring mastication; three weeks after the operation soft solids may be allowed. Nasal feeding may be ordered for the first days after the operation.

(3) **Operations on the Tongue.** Following operations on the tongue (including the insertion of radium needles), the

patient is fed through a spouted feeder with rubber tubing attached. The tubing must be put at the side of the mouth and well to the back. The mouth is irrigated before and after feeds.

Careful attention should be paid to the thorough cleansing of the spout of the feeder and the rubber tubing after use, using a small brush for the spout. The feeder and tubing should then be boiled and placed in a sterile covered bowl in readiness for the next feed.

10

Administration of Drugs: Weights and Measures: Solutions

DRUGS are substances obtained from vegetable, mineral and animal sources and used for medicinal purposes. They may be introduced into the body in various forms and by various routes. Drugs may be dispensed in liquid form as solutions, tinctures, infusions, emulsions or oils, or in solid form as pills, powders, tablets or capsules.

Drugs may be administered by mouth or parenterally, that is to say they may be introduced by other routes than the alimentary tract, such as subcutaneously, intramuscularly or intravenously. Less commonly, drugs may be introduced into the rectum, inhaled or applied to the skin or mucous membrane.

Medicines for administration by mouth must be stored in a cupboard reserved for this purpose, and substances intended for external application only must be kept in a separate cupboard.

Drugs controlled by the Dangerous Drugs Act.

The Dangerous Drugs Act controls the sale and use of substances liable to cause drug addiction. Opium and its alkaloids, notably morphine, cocaine and Indian hemp were the drugs controlled by the original Act; more recent additions are pethidine hydrochloride, methadone hydrochloride (amidone) and phenadoxone hydrochloride. These drugs may be supplied to the public only on the written prescription of a medical practitioner. Hospital wards and departments are, however, authorized to keep a stock of certain preparations, such as morphine and pethidine, but they must be ordered on a duplicate form signed by the authorized responsible person, *i.e.* the sister or charge nurse who is responsible for the safe storage of the drugs and for ensuring that they are used only in accordance with written orders of the medical staff. D.D.A. drugs must be kept in a locked cupboard reserved for the storage of these drugs the key of which is kept by the sister or charge nurse; the containers must have the words "D.D.A." written on the label. All prescriptions and order forms must be kept by the hospital for a period of two years from the date of issue.

The Poisons and Pharmacy Act

This Act controls the sale, prescribing and use of a very large range of substances which are potentially toxic or dangerous. There are sixteen schedules under the Act which list a great number of poisonous substances and the regulations to be observed in their use. The two schedules which are of particular importance in medical and hospital practice are the First and Fourth Schedules. In hospitals Schedule I can be considered as including Schedule IV drugs; they can be obtained from the pharmacist's department only on the written order of a medical officer or the sister or charge nurse of the ward or department. They must be clearly labelled Schedule I and stored in a locked cupboard. It should be noted that the toxic and addiction forming drugs controlled by the Dangerous Drugs Act are also listed on Schedule I. The usual practice with regard to storage is to have a drug cupboard for Schedule I poisons with an inner cupboard fitted with a separate lock and key for D.D.A. Drugs. It is important to remember that the "poisons cupboard" must be reserved solely for the storage of D.D.A. and Scheduled drugs.

Examples of drugs on the First and Fourth Schedule of the Poisons and Pharmacy Act are the toxic alkaloids such as atropine and hyoscine and the barbiturates.

The Therapeutic Substances (Prevention of Misuse) Act, 1956, controls substances which are capable of causing danger to the health of the community if used without proper safeguards. The form of prescription is the same as for Fourth Schedule Drugs which may only be prescribed by a medical practitioner, dentist or veterinary surgeon. Drugs controlled by this Act include antibiotics, cortisone, prednisone and isoniazid.

Each ward and department should keep a Dangerous Drugs and Poisons record book in which the patient's name, the drug, the dose, the date and the time of administration are entered and each entry signed by the nurse giving and the nurse checking the drug.

Administration of Drugs by Mouth

Rules to be observed. (1) Read the label on the bottle before removing the bottle from the shelf and again before pouring out the dose.

(2) Shake the bottle.

(3) Hold the bottle with the labelled side uppermost. A soiled label is not only unsightly, but dangerous, since it may become illegible.

(4) Remove the cork, holding it in the little finger of the left hand.

(5) Measure the dose at eye level.

(6) If there is a sediment, provide a glass rod to stir the medicine immediately before the patient takes it.

(7) Check once more to be sure that you have the right medicine, the right dose, and that you are taking it to the right patient.

(8) Give the medicine at the correct time and see that the patient takes it.

(9) If the mixture contains a drug controlled by the Dangerous Drugs Act or a Schedule 1 drug a second person should check the dose.

(10) Once poured out, the medicine should not be returned to the bottle. Medicine should never be given from an unlabelled or illegibly labelled bottle, or from an unmarked container.

Times for Administration of Medicine.—If a medicine is ordered three times a day with no other directions, it is given immediately after the three main meals of the day—*i.e.* breakfast, dinner and supper.

A medicine ordered before food is given fifteen to twenty minutes before a meal.

A medicine ordered twice a day is usually given after breakfast and supper, unless special times are stated.

A medicine ordered four-hourly is given at four-hourly intervals throughout the day and night, but special instructions should be obtained regarding waking the patient at night.

Slow-acting purgatives are given at night, quick-acting purgatives in the early morning.

General Remarks. Most medicines have an unpleasant taste, and the majority of patients can be allowed a drink of water, a piece of fruit or a sweet to take away the taste.

Holding the nose while drinking is sometimes a help, as taste depends to some extent on smell.

A medicine containing iron, stains the teeth and should be taken through a glass drinking tube or a straw. The mouth should be washed out afterwards and the teeth cleaned.

Powders are most easily swallowed if put upon the tongue and washed down with a drink of water. They may be put into a rice-paper cachet, which should be moistened with some water in a spoon, as it can then be more easily swallowed.

Pills and capsules are swallowed with a drink of water.

Oily substances are difficult to take, not only on account of the flavour, but also because of the disagreeable taste of oil in the mouth. Liquid paraffin has no distinct flavour and is fairly easy to swallow if a little soda or plain water is added. Castor oil is extremely unpleasant to take, both on account of its taste and the thickness of the oil. Infants, however, will usually take castor oil from a spoon quite readily, and older children will often take it beaten up in warm milk. For an adult patient the oil must be prepared so that the patient can drink it all at once without tasting it. One method is to warm a china measure or medicine glass in hot water; about 2 teaspoonfuls of lemon juice or mixed lemon and orange juice are poured into the measure and the prescribed dose of the oil floated on top of this. More fruit juice is poured on to the top of the oil. A slice of lemon or orange may be taken to the bedside with the dose. The patient is told to bite the piece of lemon, then swallow the dose at one gulp and bite the slice of lemon again.

The disadvantages of giving drugs by mouth are:

(1) The patient may not be able to or may refuse to swallow the dose.

(2) The drug may be only partially absorbed.

(3) It may irritate the alimentary tract, causing vomiting or acting as a purgative, so that the desired effect is lost.

Administration of Drugs by the Rectum. The drug is dissolved in about 4 oz. of normal saline or water and injected slowly at body temperature.

The following drugs may be given *per rectum*: potassium bromide, chloral, paraldehyde, bromethol. Drugs incorporated in a base of coconut butter in the form of suppositories are also introduced into the rectum, usually for their local effect.

Administration of Drugs by the Skin. The intact skin can absorb only oily substances. Apart from the ointments used in treating local conditions, inunction was at one time used as a means of introducing mercury into the body in the treatment of syphilis. Mercury has been superseded by injections of chemotherapeutic preparations and mercurial inunction in the treatment of syphilis is not now employed.

Administration of Drugs by Inhalation. Drugs given by this method may be ordered for their general effect, or for a local effect on the respiratory passages. The substance must either be in the form of a vapour or a liquid which readily volatilizes.

The anæsthetic gases and oxygen are examples of drugs exerting a general effect when inhaled.

Aromatic substances as menthol, tincture of benzoin, and pine oil may be added to steam inhalations for their local effects in the treatment of acute sinusitis or laryngitis.

Administration of Drugs by Hypodermic Injection. The drugs given by this method are usually potent drugs, of which only small amounts are required. The action of the drug is quicker than when given by mouth.

The drugs are usually dispensed in solution either in multi-dose containers or in ampoules containing a single dose. Tablets which are dissolved in sterile water for injection are also obtainable.

The usual site for a hypodermic injection is the outer aspect of the arms or of the thighs.

All glass or "record" type syringes of 1- or 2-ml. capacity and needles size 17 to 20 are used for hypodermic injections. For sterilization of syringes see pp. 129–132.

Before giving the injection it should be ascertained that the needle is not bent nor its point blunted. A bent needle may snap at the hilt when used and a blunt needle will give unnecessary pain. The nurse should also make certain that the needle fits the syringe, otherwise the fluid will leak round the joint when the injection is given. If syringes are stored in alcohol this must be expelled and the syringe washed in sterile water before use.

The nurse should place the syringe on a tray, with the needle resting on a piece of sterile gauze, together with a swab moistened with alcohol or cetrimide for cleaning the skin. A pair of sterile dressing forceps for handling the needle may be required. She should take the tray with the bottle or container and the patient's prescription sheet to a second person to be checked. The dose should be measured in the presence of the person checking it.

Solutions for hypodermic injections may be dispensed in multidose rubber-capped bottles. The bottle should be held so that the cap is not handled. After wiping the cap of the bottle with a swab moistened with alcohol, the needle should be pushed through the centre of the cap and a little air injected to facilitate the removal of the fluid. Slightly more than the required quantity of the solution should be taken up, and then, holding the syringe with the needle vertical, the piston is pushed up until the edge is on a level with the line showing the required number of minims. The exact dose should then be measured and the air expelled as just described.

When using drugs in tablet form a small amount of water should be boiled in a spoon and a convenient amount (10 to 12 minims) taken up in the syringe. The excess water in the spoon is then discarded, the tablet placed in the spoon, and the water from the syringe expelled into it. The tablet dissolves readily and the solution is drawn up into the syringe.

If the drug is in a glass ampoule, a file is required to make a mark on the neck of the ampoule where it is to be broken. The outside of the glass is washed with a swab, moistened with alcohol and, holding the ampoule in a piece of sterile gauze, the neck is then broken at the file mark.

If the patient is not familiar with the procedure, the nurse should explain to him what she is about to do and that he will feel only a very small prick. An injection made with a sharp needle is scarcely felt.

The site of the injection should be rubbed fairly vigorously with a swab moistened with alcohol, in order both to cleanse the skin and to increase the blood supply. A small piece of skin and subcutaneous tissue should be taken up between the thumb and first finger of the left hand, pulling the skin fairly taut. The needle is inserted quickly and firmly, and the piston pushed steadily down. The mop should be pressed on the skin while the needle is withdrawn. A little massage of the site with the mop will hasten the absorption of the fluid.

Among the drugs commonly given by hypodermic injection are adrenaline, atropine, hyoscine, morphine, papaveretum (Omnopon), and nikethamide (Coramine).

Administration of Drugs by Intramuscular Injection. This method is used when larger amounts are required to be injected than can be given by hypodermic injection, and is also chosen when the drug would be irritating if injected superficially. The sites usually chosen are the vastus externus muscle of the outer aspect of the thigh, the gluteal muscles of the buttock, or the deltoid muscle in the upper part of the arm. It is essential to avoid giving the injection into a blood vessel, nerve or periosteum. To ascertain that the needle is not in a vein the plunger should be withdrawn a little; if blood is drawn up into the syringe, then a vein has been punctured and the needle should be moved slightly and the plunger once more withdrawn before making the injection. When making an injection into the buttock the upper and outer quadrant should be chosen, as there is a risk of stabbing the sciatic nerve if the needle is inserted too near the sacrum. Periosteum can be avoided by giving the injection into a site where there is plenty of muscle covering the bone and by not stabbing too deeply.

The injection and the skin over the site are prepared in the manner described for the giving of hypodermic injections. The size of syringe and needles required will depend on the amount and type of the drug to be injected and on the site of the injection, *i.e.* whether or not it is necessary to penetrate deeply into the tissues, 1, 2 or 5 ml. syringes may be needed and needles 2 to $2\frac{1}{2}$ inches long.

The needle should be inserted in a more vertical direction than when giving a subcutaneous injection.

Many drugs may be given by intramuscular injection. Some common examples are liver extracts, soluble sulphonamide preparations, penicillin and streptomycin.

Sensitization Dermatitis. Dermatitis, particularly of the hands, arms and face, may occur in nurses and doctors who come into frequent contact with penicillin and streptomycin when giving injections. An investigation into this problem has shown that spraying of the antibiotic occurs when the air is expelled from the syringe and when the needle used for withdrawal of the drug from the container is changed for another needle for giving the injection. Contamination of the hands is also likely if there is a leakage at the junction of the needle and the nozzle of the syringe. In order to minimize the risk of dermatitis it is recommended that the air should be expelled from the syringe into the container before the needle is withdrawn and that the same needle should be used for giving the injection. Care should also be taken to ensure that the needle is firmly attached to the syringe. Wearing rubber gloves gives added protection and the gloves, hands and arms should be thoroughly washed under running water when the procedure is completed. The syringe and needle should also be washed under running water.

Prolonged testing has proved that the needle is not blunted by puncturing the rubber cap of the container.

Disposable Single-dose Injection Units

Disposable drug containers and injectors are available which have the advantages of providing sealed sterile equipment ready for immediate use. Further, the use of these injector units for antibiotic drugs considerably reduces the risk of sensitization dermatitis for doctors and nurses who have to give large numbers of these injections. The apparatus consists of a glass ampoule containing the solution to be injected and an inert gas and a needle protected by a glass cover. A flexible plastic envelope covers the neck of the ampoule and the hilt of the needle. The glass protecting tube is given a quick snap and removed. When the needle is inserted, the neck of the ampoule is broken through the flexible plastic tubing and the solution flows through the needle under the pressure exerted by the gas in the ampoule.

Intravenous Injection. This method of introducing drugs or fluid into the circulation is undertaken by the doctor.

The usual reasons for using this route are:

(1) When a very quick action is required in an emergency—*e.g.* cardiac and respiratory stimulants such as nikethamide, adrenaline.

(2) When the drug used would be irritating to the tissues if given intramuscularly or hypodermically—*e.g.* arsenical preparations.

(3) When large amounts are to be given as for example the intravenous administration of blood, plasma and other fluids.

(4) When it is desired to introduce a drug into the circulation for diagnostic purposes—*e.g.* diodine, indigocarmine.

(5) When it is desired to produce local clotting in the treatment of varicose veins.

Intravenous injection is also used as a route for the administration of anæsthetics such as thiopentone sodium (Pentothal).

The usual site for the injection is one of the large superficial veins on the front of the elbow.

Requirements:

The drug for injection.   If the drug has been stored in a refrigerator time must be allowed for it to reach room temperature before administration.

A sterile 10- or 20-ml. syringe.

A tourniquet or a sphygmomanometer.

A roller bandage for the patient to grip.

Sterile swabs and a sterile towel.

Instrument forceps.

Ether, surgical spirit or cetrimide.

A mackintosh.

A small gauze dressing and collodion for sealing the puncture.

A receiver for dirty swabs.

The skin should be cleaned round the site of the injection, and the tourniquet or the cuff of the sphygmomanometer placed round the arm well above the elbow and then tightened or inflated sufficiently to distend the veins.   The cuff of the sphygmomanometer is more convenient than a tourniquet, as it is easier to regulate the pressure so that the venous, but not the arterial, circulation is stopped.   Also the wide cuff of the sphygmomanometer is more comfortable for the patient than a narrow rubber tourniquet.

The patient, if able to do so, may help by gripping the roller bandage tightly or by opening and closing his fist several times.

The nurse will be required to assist by steadying the patient's arm while the needle is being inserted and by releasing the tourniquet or deflating the cuff when the needle is in the vein.

After use the syringe and needle should be cleaned at once, it is a good plan to have a bowl of cold water at hand in which they can be placed when the doctor has completed the injection.

WEIGHTS AND MEASURES

Imperial System

Measures of Mass (Weights)

Apothecaries'

1 grain (gr.)
1 scruple = 20 grains.
1 drachm = 60 grains = 3 scruples.
1 ounce = 480 grains = 8 drachms.
1 pound (lb.) = 12 ounces = 5,760 grains.

Avoirdupois

1 grain (gr.)
1 ounce (oz.) = 437·5 grains.
1 pound (lb.) = 16 ounces = 7,000 grains.

Measures of Capacity (Volumes)

1 minim (m.)
1 fluid drachm (fl. dr.) = 60 minims.
1 fluid ounce (fl. oz.) = 8 fl. dr.
1 pint   = 20 fl. oz.
1 quart   = 2 pints.
1 gallon   = 4 quarts.

Roman numerals were formerly used in prescription writing—*e.g.* I, II, III, IV. It is now recommended that Roman numerals and the ancient symbols (*e.g.* ʒ, ℥) be no longer used, and that quantities ordered should be written in arabic numerals and expressed in simple abbreviations—*e.g.* grains (gr.), ounces (oz.), fluid ounces (fl. oz.), drachms (dr.), minims (m.).

The nurse must be careful not to confuse the symbols of the Imperial and Metric systems.

Metric System

Measures of Mass (Weights)

1 milligram (mg.)$=\frac{1}{1000}$ gramme or 0·001 g.

1 centigram (cg.) $=\frac{1}{100}$ gramme or 0·01 g.

1 decigram (dg.) $=\frac{1}{10}$ gramme or 0·1 g.

1 gramme (G. or g.)=weight of 1 millilitre (ml.) of distilled water at 4° C. The accepted symbol in prescription writing is G., since gm. and grm. are likely to be confused with gr. (grain).

1 kilogram (kg.) =1,000 grammes.

Measures of Capacity (Volumes)

1 centimil (cml.) =the vol. of 1 centigram of water at 4° C.

1 decimil (dml.) =the vol. of 1 decigram of water at 4° C.

1 millilitre
or mil (ml.) =the vol. of 1 gramme of water at 4° C.

1 litre (l.) =the vol. of 1,000 grammes (1 kg.) of water at 4° C.

N.B.—The cubic centimetre (c.c.), which is approximately equal to 1 millilitre, should not be used as a unit of volume. The accepted abbreviation for "millilitre" is "ml."

Approximate Equivalencies—Imperial and Metric

Weight: Imperial to Metric

Imperial Grain	Metric Gramme	Imperial Grains	Metric Grammes
$\frac{1}{1000}$	0·00006	2	0·13
$\frac{1}{200}$	0·0003	3	0·19
$\frac{1}{100}$	0·0006	4	0·26
$\frac{1}{64}$	0·001	5	0·32
$\frac{1}{50}$	0·0013	6	0·39
$\frac{1}{40}$	0·0016	8	0·52
$\frac{1}{32}$	0·0021	10	0·65
$\frac{1}{25}$	0·0326	12	0·8
$\frac{1}{20}$	0·0032	15	1·0
$\frac{1}{16}$	0·0042	20	1·3
$\frac{1}{12}$	0·0054	30	2·0
$\frac{1}{10}$	0·0065	45	3·0
$\frac{1}{8}$	0·008	60	4·0
$\frac{1}{6}$	0·011	90	6·0
$\frac{1}{5}$	0·013	120	8·0
$\frac{1}{4}$	0·016	150	10·0
$\frac{1}{3}$	0·022	180	12·0
$\frac{1}{2}$	0·032	½ oz. (Av.)	14·2
$\frac{3}{4}$	0·049	1 oz. (Av.)	28·35
1	0·065	1 pound (Av.)	453·6
1½	0·097		

Weight: Metric to Imperial

1 kilogram = 2 lb. $3\frac{1}{4}$ oz.
500 grammes = 1 lb. $1\frac{1}{4}$ oz.
100 grammes = $3\frac{1}{2}$ oz.
25 grammes = $\frac{7}{8}$ oz. = 386 grains.
10 grammes = $\frac{1}{3}$ oz. = 154 grains.
1 gramme   = 15·4 grains.
0·5 gramme   = 7·7 grains.

Volume: Imperial to Metric

Minims	Millilitres	Fl. drachms	Millilitres
$\frac{1}{2}$	0·03	$\frac{1}{2}$	1·8
1	0·06	1	3·6
2	0·12	2	7·1
3	0·18	6	21·3
4	0·24		
5	0·3	*Fl. ounces*	*Millilitres*
6	0·4	$\frac{1}{2}$	14·2
8	0·5	1	28·4
10	0·6	2	56·8
12	0·7	4	113·7
15	0·9	5	142·1
20	1·2	6	170·5
25	1·5	8	227·5
30	1·8	10	284·2
40	2·4	20	568·4
45	2·7		
60	3·6	*Gallons*	*Litres*
90	5·3	1	4·546
120	7·1		
240	14·2		

Relations of Volume to Weight

1 minim is the volume at 16·7° C. (62° F.) of 0·911 grain of water.

1 fl. drachm is the volume at 16·7° C. (62° F.) of 54·687 grains of water.

1 fl. ounce is the measure at 16·7° C. (62° F.) of 437·5 grains of water. (Av. ounce.)

1 pint is the measure at 16·7° C. (62° F.) of 8750·0 grains of water.

Percentage Solutions

The term "per cent." is used to mean:

(*a*) Per cent. W/W = weight in weight.
(*b*) ,, ,, V/V = volume in volume.
(*c*) ,, ,, W/V = weight in volume.

Where the Imperial System of weights and measures is used, calculation of dosage presents a difficulty because

1 minim is not the volume of 1 grain of water but only of 0·911 grain. Therefore 100 grains of water measure 110 minims (accurately 109·7143) at 16·7° C. Therefore a 1 per cent. W/V solution equals 1 grain in 110 minims.

From above figures the amounts can be calculated for any quantity of a solution of any percentage.

1 per cent. solution prepared according to the metric system is equivalent to 1 gramme in 100 ml., and prepared according to the Apothecaries' System is equivalent to 1 grain in 110 minims.

The Metric System is increasingly used in prescribing and the dosage of most of the newer drugs is expressed in terms of this system. In giving approximately equivalent Metric and Imperial dosages it is usual to reckon that 1 gramme = 15 grains and 1 millilitre = 15 minims. 1 grain is taken to equal 60 milligrams.

Table of Percentage Solutions

(To nearest second decimal figure)

Per cent.	Grains per fl. oz.	Per cent.	Grains per fl. oz.
10·0	43·75	1·8	7·88
9·5	41·56	1·7	7·44
9·0	39·37	1·6	7·00
8·5	37·19	1·5	6·56
8·0	35·00	1·4	6·12
7·5	32·81	1·3	5·69
7·0	30·62	1·2	5·25
6·5	28·44	1·1	4·81
6·0	26·25	1·0	4·37
5·5	24·06	0·9	3·94
5·0	21·87	0·8	3·50
4·5	19·69	0·7	3·06
4·0	17·50	0·6	2·62
3·5	15·31	0·5	2·19
3·0	13·12	0·4	1·75
2·5	10·94	0·3	1·31
2·0	8·75	0·2	0·87
1·9	8·31	0·1	0·44

Method of Calculating Fractional Doses and of Diluting Stock Solutions

Many of the drugs given by parenteral routes, *i.e.* sub-cutaneously, intravenously and intramuscularly, are commonly dispensed in ampoules containing one therapeutic dose, *e.g.* morphine is dispensed in ampoules containing ⅙, ¼, ⅓ and ½ grain. Drugs are, however, also dispensed in rubber-capped bottles of stock solution and it may be necessary to calculate a fractional dose from the solution supplied and examples of the method employed are, therefore, given:

Examples

(1) The solution of hyoscine hydrobromide supplied is $\frac{1}{160}$ gr. in 15 minims water and the prescribed dose for a patient is $\frac{1}{100}$ grain. $\frac{1}{160}$ gr. in 15 minims = 1 gr. in 160×15 minims. Therefore $\frac{1}{100}$ gr. will be contained in $\frac{160 \times 15}{100} = 24$ minims.

(2) A solution of picrotoxin contains $\frac{1}{20}$ grain in 15 minims and the dose required is $\frac{1}{30}$ grain. $\frac{1}{20}$ gr. in 15 minims = 1 gr. in 15×20 minims. Therefore, $\frac{1}{30}$ gr. will be contained in $\frac{15 \times 20}{30}$ m. = 10 minims.

To dilute Stock Solutions of Lotions. Divide the strength of the dilution required by the strength of the stock solution to obtain the total number of parts required; one part will be stock solution, the remaining number of parts the required addition of the diluent.

Example. Stock solution of phenol lotion is 1–20 and 24 fl. oz. of a dilution of 1–120 is required.

120 divided by 20 = 6; therefore, 1 part of the 1–20 solution and 5 parts of water, *i.e.* 4 fl. oz. phenol and 20 fl. oz. water, are required.

Young's formula for calculating the proportion of the adult dose of a drug to be given to a child:

$$\left(\frac{\text{Age of child}}{\text{Age of child} + 12}\right) \times \text{adult dose.}$$

Example. The adult dose of a mixture containing bromide is 1 oz. How much of this mixture should be given to a child aged six?

$$\left(\frac{6}{6+12}\right) \times 480 \text{ minims—}i.e. \text{ 160 minims.}$$

Note. Young's formula is an approximation and should be used only with certain reservations.

Insulin Dosage

The standard strengths of insulin for injection are:

20 units per ml.
40 units per ml.
80 units per ml.

For the injection of insulin a syringe of 1 ml. capacity graduated in 20 divisions may be used and this is the type usually supplied to the patient who gives his own injections. If the insulin solution to be used is single strength, *i.e.* 20 units in each ml., then each division represents 1 unit, if it is double strength then each division is 2 units, and if it is quadruple strength each division is 4 units. Obviously the patient must be carefully instructed as to the exact amount to be drawn up into the syringe and this is particularly important if the dosage or the strength of the insulin is altered. For example, if the dose is 40 units and double strength insulin is used, then the patient must draw up 1 ml., 20 divisions; if, however, a change is made to quadruple strength and the dose remains at 40 units, then each division represents 4 units and the amount to be drawn is 0·5 ml., *i.e.* 10 divisions.

Syringes of 1 or 2 millilitre capacity are also used for the injection of insulin and these syringes may be graduated in 0·1 ml. ($\frac{1}{10}$) or 0·2 ml. ($\frac{1}{5}$).

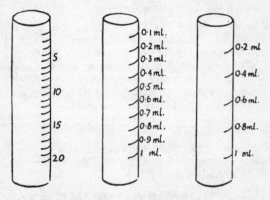

FIG. 15.—GRADUATIONS ON "INSULIN" SYRINGE AND 1 ml. SYRINGE BARRELS

Using a syringe in which each division on the barrel corresponds to 0·1 ml., and with an insulin strength of 20 units per ml., each division represents 2 units of insulin. If the strength of insulin is 40 units per ml. then each division represents 4 units of insulin, and with 80 units per ml. each division represents 8 units of insulin.

Example. The strength of the insulin to be used is 40 units per ml. and the dose ordered is 32 units.

The required dose will be $\frac{32}{40}$ ml. = 0·8 ml., and since each division on the syringe represents 4 units, the amount to be drawn up will correspond with the eighth graduation on the barrel ($\frac{32}{4} = 8$).

If each division on the syringe used represents 0·2 ml. then, using insulin in the strength of 20 units per ml., each graduation equals 4 units of insulin. If the insulin strength is 40 units per ml. each graduation equals 8 units, and with 80 units per ml. each graduation equals 16 units of insulin.

Example. Using a syringe graduated in 0·2 ml. and insulin in the strength of 80 units per ml., the dose ordered is 64 units.

The required dose will be $\frac{64}{80}$ ml. = 0·8 ml., and since each division on the syringe represents 16 units the amount to be drawn up will correspond with the fourth graduation on the barrel ($\frac{64}{16} = 4$).

Latin Words and Abbreviations used in Prescription Writing

Word or Abbreviation.	*Meaning.*
Aa, Ana (Greek preposition)	Of each.
Ad lib., Ad libitum	As much as is desired.
B.i.d., Bis in die	Twice a day.
B.P.	British Pharmacopœia.
c., Cum	With.
C., Congius	A gallon.
Cataplasma	A poultice.
Cibus	Food.
A.c., Ante cibum	Before food.
P.c., Post cibum	After food.
Collun, Collunarium	A nasal wash.
Collut., Collutorium	A mouth wash.
Collyr., Collyrium	An eye wash.
Co., Compositus	Compound.
Cras	Tomorrow.
Emplastrum	A plaster.
Flavus	Yellow.
*G, g.	Gramme.
gr., Granum, Grana	A grain, grains.
Gtt., Gutta, Guttæ	A drop, drops.
H., Hora	An hour.
Lb., libra	A pound.
Mane	In the morning.
Mist., Mistura	A mixture.
Mol., Mollis	Soft.

* Great care must be taken to distinguish between the symbols for a *gramme* and a *grain*, as mistakes can easily be made.

Abbreviations used in Prescription Writing—*cont.*

Word or Abbreviation.	*Meaning.*
Nocte	At night.
O., Octarius	A pint.
Ol., Oleum	Oil.
Om., Omnis	All, every.
O.h., Omni hora	Every hour.
O.m., Omni mane	Every morning.
O.n., Omni nocte	Every night.
†P.r.n., Pro re nata	Occasionally as need arises
Qq., Quaque	Each or every.
Qq.h., Quaque hora	Each hour.
Qq. q.h., Quaque quarta hora	Every four hours.
Q.s., Quantum sufficit	As much as is sufficient.
†S.o.s., Si opus sit	If necessary.
Ss., Semis	A half.
Stat., Statim	Immediately.
Ter.	Thrice.
T.d. or t.i.d., Ter die, ter in die	Thrice a day.
T.d.s., Ter die sumendum	To be taken three times a day.

THERMOMETRIC SCALES

Centigrade Scale

Zero, or 0° C. = temperature of melting ice at sea level (freezing point).

100° C. = temperature of steam given off water boiling under atmospheric pressure at sea level (boiling point).

Fahrenheit Scale

32° F. = temperature of melting ice at sea level (freezing point).

212° F. = temperature of steam given off water boiling under atmospheric pressure at sea level (boiling point).

Therefore the same interval of temperature is divided into 180 degrees on Fahrenheit scale (212°–32°) and 100 degrees on Centigrade scale.

$$\therefore \quad 1° \text{ F.} = \frac{100°}{180} \text{ C. or } \frac{5°}{9}\text{C.}$$

$$\therefore \quad 1° \text{ C.} = \frac{180°}{100} \text{ F. or } \frac{9°}{5}\text{F.}$$

To convert F. to C. deduct 32, multiply by 5 and divide by 9.

To convert C. to F. multiply by 9, divide by 5 and add 32.

† *P.r.n.* usually denotes that the drug may be repeated as necessary, the interval usually being stated; a drug ordered *s.o.s.* is given once only.

Thermometric Equivalents

| Centigrade to Fahrenheit. | | Fahrenheit to Centigrade. | |
Cent. degrees	Fahr. degrees	Fahr. degrees	Cent. degrees
0	32	0	—17·8
4	39·2	4	—15·5
8	46·4	8	—13·3
10	50	10	—12·2
20	68	20	— 6·6
30	86	30	— 1·1
40	104	40	4·4
50	122	50	10
60	140	60	15·5
70	158	70	21
80	176	80	27
90	194	90	32
100	212	100	37·8

11

Sterilization: Principles and Practical Application

STERILIZATION in the surgical sense means the process whereby a substance or body is rendered free from living organisms, and under this term are included various methods of killing bacteria and other micro-organisms.

All instruments, utensils and dressings used in the conduct of surgical dressings and other procedures for which aseptic precautions are necessary must be sterile and must then be handled only by a person with surgically clean gloved hands or with sterile forceps.

The word "asepsis" implies the absence of micro-organisms, while "antisepsis" (against sepsis) usually implies the use of chemical disinfectants to kill micro-organisms. Aseptic precautions in a ward or theatre imply that all dressings and appliances are sterile and that there is no risk of contaminating the wound and while similar precautions are taken with septic cases, additional antiseptic precautions may be taken to prevent spread of infection.

In common practice all articles that can be sterilized by heat are treated in this way; when this method is not practicable, then chemical disinfectants are used.

It cannot be too strongly emphasized that all dressing utensils and materials must be kept free from contamination with gross dirt even if they are to be sterilized before use and also that aseptic precautions are as necessary in dealing with an infected wound as with a clean one. The danger to the patient is increased if a fresh infection is introduced.

Sterilization by Physical Means

Heat kills all forms of bacterial life, although those organisms which can take on a protective spore formation can withstand a higher temperature for a longer period than the less resistant, or vegetative, forms.

Boiling for two minutes in plain water, or water containing 2 per cent. sodium carbonate, has been shown by bacteriological tests to be an efficient means of sterilization suitable for most instruments, glass, rubber and enamel articles. The addition of sodium carbonate (washing soda) to the boiling water enhances the lethal effect of the heat and also prevents rusting of metal instruments. To allow a margin of safety five minutes may be taken as the standard time for sterilization by boiling. Elastic gum articles which are damaged by prolonged exposure to heat are usually boiled for two minutes only. Materials which are poor conductors of heat, such as linen, or silk thread wound on reels, are boiled for a longer period than five minutes to allow the heat to penetrate to the inner layers, thirty minutes is a suitable time for these materials. Although five minutes' boiling will kill most organisms, some spore-forming organisms, notably those of tetanus and gas gangrene will only be killed by prolonged boiling or by exposure to high temperatures in an autoclave. Contaminated articles may be subjected to a period of boiling of one hour and then allowed to cool in order to allow any resistant spores to change to the vegetative form; a second boiling for one hour then kills any organisms that survived the first process.

Although, as has been stated, five minutes may be taken as a safe standard time for most articles sterilized by boiling, the efficiency of this method depends on strict observance of certain rules:

    (i) The water must be boiling for the full five minutes. The addition of a large number of cold instruments or bowls will reduce the temperature. The timing, therefore, must not start until the water in the sterilizer has again reached boiling point.

    (ii) The sterilizer must contain sufficient water to cover all the articles completely.

    (iii) No additional articles must be put in the sterilizer after the timing of the five-minute period has begun and the lid of the sterilizer must be properly closed throughout the operation.

    (iv) Articles such as bowls, gallipots and receivers must not be stacked tightly one inside the other because this creates air pockets which interfere with the penetration of heat.

(v) Sterilizers and equipment must be maintained in good condition. Scale formation due to minerals in the water roughens the surface of both the sterilizer and the articles boiled in it.

Sterlization by Steam under Pressure (Autoclaving)

Steam kills organisms by coagulation of the cell protein provided that certain factors are present; the steam must be under pressure, dry and saturated. With these conditions fulfilled steam will condense when it meets a cooler surface, *i.e.* the articles in the autoclave, and the latent heat released on condensation will penetrate the material and kill any organisms present. Autoclaving at a pressure of 20 lbs. per square inch (above atmospheric pressure) and a temperature of 125° C. (260° F.) for twenty minutes is an efficient method of sterilizing fabrics (such as gowns and dressing materials), instruments and bowls. Rubber is damaged by exposure to high temperatures and such articles as rubber gloves are therefore usually subjected to autoclaving a lower temperature and pressure, such as 15 lbs. pressure and a temperature of 121° C. (250° F.) for ten minutes.

The times given refer to the "holding time" after the required temperature has been reached, the total time required for the full process after loading the autoclave depends on the type of apparatus used, in modern high-vacuum sterilizers the time required for the penetration of steam and raising of the temperature in the sterilizing chamber is very much less than in the older types of apparatus. It is essential for effective sterilization that all materials should be loosely packed in their containers.

In addition to recording the temperature and pressure readings during the sterilization process, proof of effective sterilization can be gained by burying control tubes in the centre of the containers, these tubes contain an indicator which changes colour when the correct temperature has been reached. Bacteriological tests are also usually carried out at regular intervals.

Pasteurization. This term is applied to a method most commonly used to destroy the organisms present in milk. The milk is exposed to a temperature of 145° F. to 150° F. for thirty minutes. It is then rapidly cooled to 55° F. or lower. This heat is sufficient to kill the ordinary forms of bacterial life likely to be present in milk, and in particular the tubercle bacillus, without altering the taste or composition of the milk. "Flash method" of pasteurization where the milk is brought to a temperature of 161° F. for 15 seconds is now commonly employed.

Dry Heat. Hot air at a temperature of 300° F. or 150° C., applied for one hour will kill all organisms. This method is not suitable for dressings or for some instruments, but is used for sterilizing laboratory glassware, such as test tubes, flasks, syringes. Infra-red rays are also used to heat ovens for sterilization by dry heat.

Other physical agents in addition to heat will destroy bacteria, but have not a very wide practical application.

Cold. Most organisms will survive exposure to very low temperatures but will not multiply. A practical application of this is the preservation of foodstuffs in cold storage.

Light. Direct sunlight kills many bacteria including the tubercle bacillus. The active agent is the ultra-violet radiation and these rays have been used to sterilize milk and water.

Drying. Moisture is as important to most bacterial cells as it is to tissue cells and removal of water will kill the cell. In certain circumstances, however, some bacteria can survive drying for considerable periods and are therefore likely to be present in dust. Examples are pyogenic organisms, diphtheria bacillus and the *Mycobacterium tuberculosis* in pus and sputum.

Gamma Radiation. This agent is not at present in general use but may in the future become increasingly important.

Chemical Disinfectants

It is essential that the nurse should understand the necessary conditions for the effective use of these agents, otherwise chemical disinfection may be quite useless and may even be dangerous if it gives rise to a false sense of security.

(1) To be efficient the disinfectant must be sufficiently strong and must be allowed to act for a sufficient length of time.

(2) With very few exceptions the disinfectant must be in solution; dry powders have very little effect.

(3) The disinfecting power of the agent varies with the

number of organisms present; highly infected material is difficult to disinfect efficiently.

(4) The disinfecting power of the agent is to a certain extent dependent upon the nature of the medium containing the organisms—*e.g.* the germicidal power is lowered in the presence of pus since in this medium many of the organisms are inside the dead leucocytes and it is difficult for the disinfectant to reach them.

(5) As a general rule it may be stated that disinfectant solutions are more effective hot than cold.

(6) Spore-forming bacteria and the acid-fast group (of which the *Mycobacterium tuberculosis* is the most important member) are much more resistant to the action of liquid disinfectants than they are to the action of heat.

(7) Disinfection usually proceeds more rapidly in an acid than in an alkaline medium.

Principal Groups of Chemical Disinfectants

A great many chemical substances are in use as disinfectants or antiseptics, many of them under proprietary names. The terms "bactericide" and "bacteriostatic", the former referring to substances which kill bacteria, and the latter to substances which inhibit bacterial growth, more accurately define the action of certain agents such as antibiotics than the words "disinfectant" and "antiseptic." At the end of this chapter a list of the commoner disinfectants, antiseptics and lotions will be found, with some notes on their particular uses.

Oxidizing and Reducing Agents. Hydrogen peroxide in the presence of organic matter readily yields oxygen and in so doing acts as a mechanical cleansing agent removing pus and debris from a wound or cavity.

Potassium permanganate is an oxidizing agent with deodorant properties. Sulphur dioxide and formalin are reducing agents which alter the nature of the bacterial cell by removing oxygen.

Halogens. These substances are a group of non-metallic elements including chlorine, iodine and bromine, the first two, chlorine and iodine, having very wide uses as disinfectants.

The chief chlorine compounds used are eusol, Dakin's

solution, chloramine and electrolytic sodium hypochlorite. These solutions liberate free chlorine which combines with proteins in the tissues and in bacterial cells. The solution has a cleansing as well as a disinfectant action since the protein of necrotic tissue and sloughs is dissolved and washed away. Iodine, like chlorine, has the power of combining with proteins. It is relatively insoluble in water but will dissolve in a solution of potassium iodide. The commonly used preparation "tincture of iodine" (Weak Solution of Iodine, B.P.) is a $2\frac{1}{2}$ per cent. solution with potassium iodine in alcohol.

Salts of Heavy Metals. These substances are first adsorbed on to the surface of the bacteria and then penetrate the organisms and kill them. The bactericidal power of most of these chemicals is, however, reduced in the presence of serum and other organic matter. Water-soluble mercurial salts, in low concentrations, are effective disinfectants for many purposes but they are irritating to the skin, tarnish metals and become relatively inactive in the presence of blood, pus and other organic matter, such as excreta. Perchloride of mercury is one of the oldest of the mercurial disinfectants and is the one in which the disadvantages just mentioned are most marked. Compounds containing very small amounts of mercury, phenylmercuric acetate and phenylmercuric nitrate, are suitable for chemical sterilization of some delicate instruments such as cystoscopes of the non-boilable type. Oxycyanide of mercury is another example of a mercurial disinfectant.

Cresol and Phenol Disinfectants. Carbolic acid is well known as the disinfectant introduced into surgical practice by Lord Lister. It is feebly acid in watery solution, but has a marked caustic action. A 5 per cent. solution will kill all vegetative bacteria and most spores in one hour; a 1 per cent. solution will kill most non-sporing organisms in ten minutes. Tar acid preparations (containing phenol, cresols, etc.) in the form of black disinfectant fluids, such as Cyllin, and white disinfectant fluids, such as Izal and Jeyes fluid, are specially suitable where large quantities of the solution are needed, as, for example, disinfecting excreta, bed-pans and linen. Their disadvantages are that they are sticky and there may be some difficulty in rinsing and cleaning utensils afterwards, also the black fluids may stain linen. Lysol is a soapy solution of

6*

cresol containing 25 per cent. soap. It is more expensive than crude phenol preparations and should be used with economy. All Cresol and phenol preparations are potentially dangerous poisons even in dilute solution.

Chlorine derivatives of cresol and xylenol, chlorocresol and chloroxylenol, are less caustic than carbolic acid or lysol. Two examples of these preparations are solution of Chloroxylenol B.P. and the proprietary substance Dettol.

Coal Tar and Aniline Dyes. The flavine group of dyes is well known in surgical practice. Formerly acriflavine was the preparation most frequently employed, proflavine is, however, more easily prepared and less irritating to the tissues than acriflavine. The flavine dyes have a specific action on staphylococci and streptococci and their activity is not decreased by the presence of serum. 5-Aminoacridine is a newer addition to the series and is practically non-staining. Aniline dyes such as brilliant green and gentian violet are used in the form of skin paints.

Cationic Detergents. These solutions of which Cetrimide and CTAB are examples have a detergent action removing grease and with it dirt and bacteria. They are not compatible with soap. Detergents are used for the cleansing of the hands, and of the skin of operation sites and for cleansing wounds. Other antiseptic and cleansing agents with a wide range of application are benzalkonium chloride (Roccal), chlorhexidine (Hibitane) and domiphen bromide (Bradosol).

Bacteriostatics which can be Administered Internally. These are chemotherapeutic and antibiotic substances.

The Sulphonamides. These substances may be administered orally or parenterally, or they may be applied locally to damaged tissue. Prontosil was the first of the group to be used, but was soon displaced by sulphanilamide, which may be looked on as the parent substance of all sulphonamides. These are active against many strains of pyogenic streptococci and are also useful in the treatment of infections of the urinary tract.

Sulphapyridine is more effective than sulphanilamide in the treatment of pneumococcal, gonococcal and meningococcal infections but has been replaced by sulphadiazine, sulphathiazole, and sulphamerazine which are active against these organisms and less toxic than sulphapyridine. Sulphaguanidine and succinyl sulphathiazole are two varieties of sulphonamides which are not readily absorbed from the alimentary tract and when given by mouth a high concentration of the drug in the intestinal tract can be obtained. These preparations are therefore used in the treatment of intestinal infections.

Isonicotinic Acid Hydrazide and Para-aminosalicylic Acid. These two chemotherapeutic drugs are used in the treatment of tuberculosis, usually in conjunction with an antibiotic, streptomycin.

Sulphone Compounds. These drugs are allied to the sulphonamides and are used in the treatment of leprosy. Dapsone and solapsone tablets are examples of sulphone preparations.

Antibiotic Substances. *Penicillin* was the first of an ever-growing list of antibiotics, *i.e.* drugs prepared from living organisms. It is obtained from the mould *Penicillium notatum*. It may be applied locally, as a cream, given by intra-muscular or intravenous injection, or by mouth. Penicillin for injection is prepared as a solution of crystalline penicillin (benzylpenicillin) and as procaine penicillin. Penicillin is given orally in the form of tablets of phenoxymethyl penicillin (penicillin-V).

Streptomycin is effective against a number of micro-organisms which are insensitive to penicillin, it is used in the treatment of tuberculosis, including miliary tuberculosis and tuberculous meningitis.

Chlortetracycline (Aureomycin), *oxytetracycline* (Terramycin) and *tetracycline* are antibiotics with similar properties which are effective in the treatment of some penicillin-resistant infections.

Chloramphenicol is used in the treatment of intestinal infections, especially typhoid fever. Although it is effective in the treatment of other infections its use is restricted because of its tendency to produce aplastic anæmia.

Erythromycin is another antibiotic used in the treatment of staphylococcal infections which are resistant to penicillin.

Information regarding progress in the knowledge and use of antibiotics should be frequently sought by the nurse. New products are continually undergoing trial, and she should keep herself particularly informed as to their modes of administration and the precautions to be observed in their use.

Cleansing and Sterilization of Instruments, Dressing Utensils and Materials

Instruments.   Most metal instruments can be boiled for five minutes in water containing 2 per cent. sodium carbonate. Sharp instruments may also be boiled if they are wrapped so as to prevent contact of the sharp edges with the sides of the sterilizer during the process.   An alternative method for scalpels and knives is to immerse them for 20 minutes in a disinfectant solution such as lysol or chloroxylenol, 1 part to 4 parts spirit.   The instruments will require to be rinsed in spirit and sterile water before use.   After boiling or chemical sterilization instruments are usually dished dry into sterile trays or boxes covered with a properly fitting lid. Instruments may be sterilized in the autoclave.   Although this is not a method at present commonly used for the ordinary ward equipment, it is increasingly employed in operating theatres and in central sterile supply departments.

Particularly delicate instruments call for special methods of sterilization and the nurse should ascertain the method to be adopted in each case; some cystoscopes, for example, are boilable and may be placed in the perforated metal box in which they are stored in a sterilizer containing warm water which is brought up to boiling point and allowed to boil for five minutes.   Other types of cystoscopes and endoscopes of various types are damaged by boiling and are sterilized in a formalin cabinet, or in a solution such as 1–10,000 phenyl mercuric nitrate or Hibitane 1 per cent. for twenty minutes.   The telescopes and sheaths of cystoscopes require special treatment; valves and irrigating nozzles may be boiled for five minutes.

After use instruments are washed in cold water and then scrubbed in hot soapy water using a brush kept for the purpose.   They should then be boiled for five minutes and afterwards dried.   Joints and grooves require special care both in cleaning and drying.   Stainless steel instruments need no other treatment except periodic oiling of the joints.

Glass Articles.—*e.g.* catheters, glass connections and syringes.

If these articles cannot be sterilized in a hot air oven they can be boiled, but should not be plunged straight into boiling water.   They may be warmed in hot water first, placed in a sterilizer and gradually brought to the boil.   They are boiled for five minutes. To reduce the risk of breakage they should not be boiled with other articles, especially heavy instruments.

After boiling and before use glass articles should be inspected for cracks or chips.

Plastic Instruments. Some instruments, especially those for diagnostic purposes, are now made with plastic parts which require special care in sterilization. "Coldlite" auriscopes, diagnostic sets and rectal and vaginal speculæ are examples of these. "Coldlite" instruments of clear plastic with metal attachments can be boiled for five minutes in plain water, but must be wrapped to prevent scratching. These instruments should never be sterilized by immersion in phenol, lysol, or any other acid disinfectant, nor should they be allowed to come into contact with instruments which have been so treated, as any trace of these disinfectants will cloud the transparent plastic. Methylated or surgical spirit will also cause discoloration. Plastic instruments cannot be autoclaved. Cetrimide, 1 per cent. solution may be used, but instruments should not be kept continuously in such a solution and should be washed and dried as quickly as possible after use. The lamps of any illuminated instruments must be removed before boiling; they may be cleaned when necessary by wiping with spirit, but immersion in spirit or any solution will weaken the cement.

Sterilization of Syringes

Two main types of syringes are in use for the injection of drugs and for the withdrawal of blood or for aspiration of pus or fluid. These are the "Record" type, which are partly glass and partly metal, and the all-glass type. Syringes should preferably be sterilized by heat. Chemical disinfectants are not recommended for this purpose for several reasons, the action of the chemical is often slow and the disinfectant cannot with certainty be assumed to have penetrated into all the crevices of the syringe; traces of the disinfectant remaining in the syringe may damage or alter the solution to be injected. The rinsing of the syringe after removal from the disinfectant is a possible source of danger, sterile water is readily contaminated once the container is opened; therefore, unless an autoclaved and previously unopened bottle can be provided for each rinsing, there is a possibility of contaminating the syringe and its contents. Drawing alcohol through a syringe before use as a means of sterilization has been demonstrated to be ineffective. Immersion of the syringe in 70 to 75 per cent. alcohol for five minutes is considered safe if the all-glass syringe is used. This method can be used, for example, for a diabetic patient's injection of insulin, provided that the syringe is washed well before the immersion and when it is rinsed after removal from spirit, precautions are taken to ensure that the water used for this purpose is freshly sterilized.

The best method of sterilization for all-glass syringes is by hot air at a temperature of 160° C. (320° F.) for one hour, this exposure will kill vegetative and spore forms of bacteria. The syringe can be assembled before sterilization and placed in a glass or metal container. Needles are also best sterilized with the syringes in the hot air oven. The containers must be efficiently sealed, and for this purpose thin aluminium foil is suitable. Sterilization may be carried out by autoclaving for twenty minutes at a pressure of 20 lb. and a temperature of 120° C. but penetration of the steam to all parts of the syringe is doubtful if the syringe is assembled before sterilization. It is also not possible to be seen that the syringe will be dry after autoclaving.

Although glass and metal syringes which will stand high temperatures are now available in some types the cement in the glass-metal seal of the nozzle may melt at high temperatures. Boiling in the ward sterilizer may be used for these syringes but cannot be relied upon to kill spores and is, therefore, not a guarantee that the syringe is in actual fact sterile, but it is stated that accidents due to contamination with spore-forming organisms are rare and the method can be considered reasonably safe. The syringe must be taken apart for sterilization as the rapid expansion of the metal piston when heated will crack the glass barrel if the syringe is assembled before boiling. A piece of lint should be placed on the tray of the sterilizer and the sterilizer filled to a sufficient level with warm (but not hot) water. The lint protects the points of the needles and also prevents the glass of the syringe from being broken against the metal base of the sterilizer. The water is brought to boiling point and the syringe boiled for five minutes. It is then lifted out in the tray of the sterilizer, drained of water and transferred with sterile instrument forceps to a sterile bowl or box with a well-fitting lid.

If a sterilizer is not available, as for example in home nursing, the syringe may be boiled in a small saucepan with a lid. When the syringe has boiled for five minutes the water can be drained off and the syringe left in the saucepan covered by the lid until it is required. Lint should not in this case be used as it will prevent the syringe from drying when the water is drained off. The addition of soda to the water in the sterilizer is recommended for the sterilization of instruments but not for the boiling of syringes, because residual alkalinity of the syringe may affect the material to be injected. In districts where the tap water is very hard the syringes may become coated with chalk which may make the markings difficult to read and cause the syringe parts to fit badly. In such cases it is advisable to use softened or distilled water in the sterilizer. Syringes with plastic pistons are now made and it is stated by the manufacturers that they can be sterilized without damage by boiling, autoclaving or by hot air.

All syringes should be washed after use in warm soapy water, using a bottle brush for the barrel, and then rinsed in clean water before drying. Infected syringes, *i.e.* those used for withdrawal of blood or for aspirating pus, should be washed immediately after use in a solution of cold disinfect-ant, a suitable one is 2 per cent. lysol, before washing in soapy water. Syringes used for these purposes should be kept separate from those used for injections.

The needle should be left attached and the fluid drawn through the syringe and expelled several times. It is essential that the washing out of the syringe should be done at once and that the disinfectant solution should be cold, otherwise the syringe nozzle or the needle may be clogged.

If several similar syringes are being washed and assembled together it is necessary to see that pistons are fitted to the right barrels, slight differences in individual syringes of the same capacity occur and, for correct fitting, identification numbers may be engraved on both barrel and piston. In order to ensure smooth working of the all-glass syringe the piston may be lightly oiled with liquid paraffin before being assembled. Many hospitals now operate a central syringe service which is under the direction of the hospital path-ologist. The cleaning, servicing and sterilization of syringes is carried out by technicians and the wards and departments collect their supplies once or twice daily.

Rubber Articles. These may be boiled in plain water without soda.

Rubber gloves should be examined for punctures before sterilization. They may then be placed in a bag with a small metal weight, so that they remain below the surface of the water, and boiled for five minutes. Filling the gloves with water also acts as a weight.

Gloves, however, are usually sterilized in the autoclave. After inspection the gloves are powdered, wrapped in gauze with a layer separating each glove, and packed in a drum with a small envelope containing powder. Separate drums may be used for the various sizes of gloves in use, or the package may be marked with the size of the gloves that it contains. After use rubber gloves are well washed on both sides with soap and water. If they have been used for a septic case they should be allowed to soak for one hour in 1–40 lysol solution before washing. They should be rinsed, boiled and then dried on a towel. Before being put away they should be inspected for punctures and powdered on both sides.

Rubber gloves are damaged by contact with dry heat such as a radiator, by grease and by acids.

Rubber tubing after use should be cleaned with cold water, then with hot soapy water and afterwards rinsed. Care must be taken to flush the inside thoroughly.

After boiling, the tubing should be hung over a rail to drain. When put away it should be loosely coiled, avoiding kinking.

Rubber catheters after use should be cleaned by running cold water through from both ends, afterwards washing and rinsing in cold water. They are then boiled for five minutes, dried outside and placed on a towel or hung up until completely dry inside. Stiffened rubber (Tieman's) male catheters are sterilized by the same method as soft rubber.

Polythene Tubing. Plastic polythene tubing can be used in place of rubber and also for intravenous or intrathecal cannulæ. The tubing can be obtained in three sizes. It is sterilized for use by boiling. As it is inexpensive, it is discarded after use.

Elastic Gum. Elastic gum instruments such as catheters

and bougies need very careful handling and sterilization because the smooth surface is easily cracked and roughened. If this occurs the catheter must be discarded, as it is likely to damage the delicate lining of the urethra. Bougies and ureteric catheters made of elastic gum may be sterilized by the same methods used for elastic gum catheters.

Two methods of sterilization are:

1. The catheters are wrapped in old linen tied either end with a length of tape or placed in a bag. They are then immersed in boiling water for two minutes, removed by the tapes or bag (not by grasping the catheters with forceps), and placed in a sterile dish or jar containing cold sterile water to stiffen them.

2. The catheters may be placed in a special airtight jar or cabinet containing paraform tablets which evolve formaldehyde gas. Twenty-four hours are required for sterilization by this method. When removed from the jar the catheters should be placed in a dish of sterile water for rinsing, as formaldehyde is irritating.

If a cabinet is available in which the paraform tablets can be heated, the process goes on much more quickly and sterilization may be complete in thirty minutes.

After use the catheters should be washed in the same way as glass and rubber catheters. They should be dried on the outer surface and left on a towel until completely dry before being put away.

It seems likely that plastic materials such as polythene will increasingly replace elastic-gum catheters and bougies.

Dressing Materials. Cotton wool, gauze, gamgee tissue and cellulose are sterilized by steam under pressure in the autoclave.

Dressing materials can be obtained cut ready for sterilization and in a variety of sizes and shapes. If this task is carried out by the nurse in the ward the cutting and packing should be done on a clean towel with clean hands.

Gauze is usually folded so that there are no raw edges. For theatre mops the gauze is made up into squares of different sizes and the edges may be sewn.

Swabs are made of wool rolled and cut into suitable sizes or of wool covered with gauze.

The dressings may be made up into packets and put into drums or other containers. Drums are lined with lint or brown paper. Separate packs containing sufficient material for one dressing or procedure may be used. Mass packing of dressing materials in one container involves a risk of contamination and may also encourage wasteful use of dressings. In any event the drum should not be tightly packed as the steam may then not permeate all the contents.

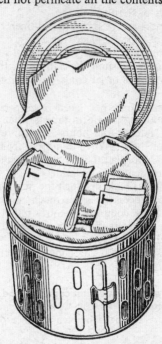

FIG. 16.—LOOSELY PACKED DRUM: STEAM CAN REACH ALL CONTENTS

For theatre use it is more usual to pack one type of article in one drum—*e.g.* swabs in one drum, gowns in another, towels in another, and so on. The perforations at the sides or top of the drum are opened just before the drum is put in the autoclave, so that the steam can penetrate. When removed from the autoclave the perforations are immediately closed.

Recently a nylon film has been introduced under the name of "Portex Autoclave Film." This is supplied in a tubular form which can be cut to any desired length and forms a container sealed at either end when the articles for sterilization have been packed. The material can be autoclaved

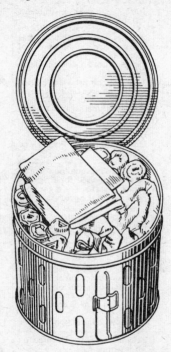

FIG. 17.—TIGHTLY PACKED DRUM: STEAM CANNOT READILY PENETRATE

as it is permeable to steam, although giving complete protection against external contamination after sterilization.

Suggestions for Further Reading

Prevention of Cross Infection in Hospitals. Medical Research Council Memorandum No. 11.

Sterilization Practice in Six Hospitals. Nuffield Provincial Hospital Trust.

The Planning and Organization of Central Syringe Services. Nuffield Provincial Hospital Trust.

Staphylococcal Infections in Hospital. Ministry of Health. H.M. Stationery Office.

Disinfectants, Antiseptics and Lotions

Substance	Uses	Strength
Alcohol.	Storing surgical instruments after sterilization. Alcohol is expensive and substitutes are available for this purpose, *e.g.* Solution of borax and formaldehyde. Alcohol is not an efficient sterilizing agent.	90–95 per cent.
Surgical spirit and industrial methylated spirit.	Cleansing of the skin, *e.g.* of operation area (spirit removes grease and with it dirt), cleaning instruments and utensils especially glass ware.	60–75 per cent.
Benzalkonium Chloride (Roccal).	Disinfection of skin. Disinfection of linen and utensils.	1 in 10 solution. 1 in 40 solution.
Boric acid.	Mild antiseptic and non-irritating lotion used for irrigating mucous surfaces, *e.g.* the conjunctiva of the eye. Boric acid powder is a component of dusting powders.	Saturated solution (4 per cent.) diluted as required for use ½ or ¼ strength.
Chloroxylenol and similar preparations, *e.g.* Dettol and Osyl.	These preparations are less irritating and less caustic than phenol or cresol, they can be used undiluted on the skin if allowed to dry uncovered. Used for skin preparation before operation or in obstetric cases. Antiseptic hand lotion.	Undiluted or 30 per cent. solution. 1-40 to 1-100.
Chlorhexidine (Hibitane).	Skin disinfection. Disinfection of instruments.	1 in 100 solution or weaker.
Chlorine, in the form of hypochlorite solutions, *e.g.* eusol, Electrolytic hypochlorite (Milton).	As a dressing or irrigating lotion in the treatment of sloughing or infected tissues.	
Cetrimide (Cetyltrimethyl ammonium bromide)	Cleansing the skin. Cleaning utensils.	1 per cent. solution.
Cresol in soap solution—lysol.	Disinfectant lotion for instrument jars. Disinfecting linen and other fabrics.	1 in 40 solution. 1-80 (½ fluid oz. to water 2 pints) if linen is left for at least 6 hours.

Disinfectants, Antiseptics and Lotions—*cont.*

Substance	Uses	Strength
Domiphen bromide (Bradosol).	Disinfection of Instruments. Cleansing wounds and irrigations.	1 in 500 solution (or weaker).
Flavine group, acriflavine, proflavine, euflavine and 5-aminoacridine.	These dyes are used in the treatment of wounds and as antiseptics on the skin. They may be combined with sterile liquid paraffin as an oily dressing.	1-1,000 solution in water or spirit. (Proflavine is not soluble in spirit.)
Formaldehyde and formalin(a solution of formaldehyde in water).	For disinfecting articles which cannot be treated with steam, *e.g.* books and leather articles, for fumigation of rooms.	If used as a spray, 8 ounces of formalin to 1 gallon of water for every 400 square feet of surface.
Paraform tablets, these disintegrate slowly liberating formaldehyde.	For the sterilization and storage of gum-elastic articles and endoscopes.	
Liquor boracis et formaldehydi.	A solution of formaldehyde with borax and phenol used for storing sterile surgical instruments.	
Hydrogen peroxide.	Used for the irrigation of wounds and cleaning septic mouth conditions. Is non-poisonous and in the presence of organic matter readily liberates oxygen and helps in the separation of sloughs.	Stock solutions contain either 10 or 20 volumes of available oxygen. Diluted with warm water, as required for use, in 2·5, 5 or 10 volumes.
Iodine.	Used for skin preparation, it is more penetrating than most skin paints especially if the skin is dry.	"Weak tincture of iodine," 2·5 per cent.
Mercurial preparations: Phenylmercuric nitrate.	Used for sterilizing certain instruments, *e.g.* the telescopes and sheaths of non-boilable cystoscopes; for preserving fluids and suspensions prepared for parenteral injection.	1-10,000 solution
	For skin preparation.	1-3,000 to 1-1,500.
	As a vaginal douche for non-specific infections.	1-3,000.
	For mycotic infections.	0·05 to 0·1 per cent. in a water soluble ointment base.

Disinfectants, Antiseptics and Lotions—*cont.*

Substance	Uses	Strength
Phenol (carbolic acid).	Liquefied phenol, carbolic acid, Poisonous and corrosive, if splashed on the skin should be swabbed off at once with methylated or surgical spirit.	
	Disinfecting linen, crockery and sanitary utensils.	5 per cent., 1-20.
	Disinfecting excreta.	10 per cent. for one hour.
Crude phenolic disinfectants, *i.e.* "black" and "white" disinfecting fluids, *e.g.* Jeyes fluid, Cyllin, Izal, etc.	Disinfecting excreta.	1-10 solution mixed with excreta for two hours.
	Disinfecting linen, "white" fluids should be used for this purpose as the "black" disinfectants may stain linen.	1-160 solution for 12 hours.
	Scrubbing floors, laboratory or sluice room benches, etc.	1-160 solution.
	For local pollution of floors, *e.g.* with sputum.	Swab with 1-5 solution.
Silver salts: Silver nitrate.	Used as an astringent and antiseptic irrigating solution, especially for application, to mucous surfaces. In the form of a solid stick it is used as a caustic.	0·02 to 2 per cent. solution.
Silver protein compounds.	These are less irritating to the tissues than silver nitrate, the official compound is Argentoproteinum B.P., containing about 8 per cent. of silver. Protargol is a similar compound.	0·25 to 1 per cent. solution.
	Argyrol is a preparation containing silver in non-ionizable form and is used in stronger solutions.	10 to 25 per cent.
Sodium chloride solutions. Normal saline (Physiological Solution of Sodium Chloride B.P.).	Used for bathing and irrigating wounds and cavities: for rectal, subcutaneous and intravenous injection.	0·9 per cent. sodium chloride in water.
Hypertonic salt solution.	In the treatment of wounds as baths or irrigations.	5-10 per cent. solution.

12

The Conduct of Surgical Dressings

THE particular needs of individual cases and the practice of surgeons in different hospitals will naturally necessitate variations in the setting of dressing trolleys and the conduct of dressings. The methods described here are based on the recommendations of the Medical Research Council's Memorandum "The Prevention of 'Hospital' Infection of Wounds." The Memorandum states that the definite incidence of hospital infection revealed by bacteriological studies conclusively indicated defects in the current aseptic technique. The chief sources of wound infection are bacteria in the air, either present in dust or in infected droplets from the mouths and noses of ward occupants and staff, and bacteria present on hands, dressings, instruments or in lotions. The Memorandum summarizes the principles which should be understood and practised. These are:

1. During the period that dressings are in progress precautions should be taken to keep the number of bacteria in the air as low as possible. Domestic activities, sweeping and bed-making, should be completed at least one hour before starting dressings. Floors may be oiled to prevent dust from rising during sweeping. Where space is available a treatment room large enough to accommodate a patient in his bed and the necessary equipment will enable such procedures to be carried out with greater safety of the patient and less disturbance of the ward routine than is the case if all procedures have to be carried out at the bedside. Masks are usually worn by all persons concerned in the conduct of surgical dressings. The mask consists of layers of muslin; a sheet of cellophane inserted between two muslin layers forms a mask which is impervious, but light in weight. "Disposable" paper masks are also available and are suitable for use over short periods. Masks should

be worn only when performing the duties which demand their use, *e.g.* when surgical operations, dressings or treatment are being carried out, when attending on patients particularly susceptible to infection, such as infants, or for the protection of the wearer when attending to patients suffering from open pulmonary tuberculosis or other infectious diseases. Masks should be removed when the duties requiring them are completed. The cellophane layer is discarded the muslin mask then placed in a bowl of disinfectant, such as lysol 1–80 and later washed and boiled.

Wards should be closed to all unnecessary traffic unless dressings can be carried out in a treatment room adjacent to the ward.

2. Hands, whether wet or dry, scrubbed or unscrubbed, are to be regarded in all circumstances as dirty, and should not be allowed to come into contact with wounds or any material directly applied to wounds. If special types of dressings cannot be managed with forceps sterile gloves should be worn.

3. Wounds should be kept covered except during the actual dressing procedure and the period for which they are then exposed should be the shortest possible. The skin around the wound should be treated with the same care as the wound itself.

4. It is easier to keep articles sterile if they are dry. Instruments after sterilization should be dished dry into sterile enamel boxes with lids or into covered bowls. Bacteria are more readily washed into a wound from wet hands and from wet instruments than from dry ones.

5. Precautions must not be relaxed when dealing with wounds that are already infected.

Preparation of the Dressing Trolley. The dressing trolley should be washed with soap and water and dried before being laid. It must be cleaned and relaid for each dressing. Fig. 18 shows a trolley set with sterile equipment on the upper shelf and unsterile equipment on the lower shelf.

Sterilized Dressings and Towels. These are packed in drums or other containers, and it is recommended that individual packets should be used in preference to bulk packaging which necessitates the passage of the same container from one dressing to another and its constant re-

opening. Sterile towels are needed to surround the area of
the wound but they are not necessary as trolley covers and
they should not be used to cover sterile articles or as temporary dressings since they are very easily displaced.

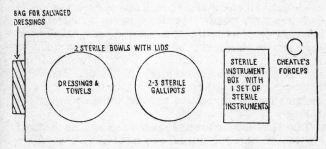

Top Shelf—sterile equipment

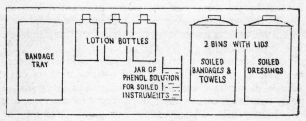

Bottom Shelf—unsterile equipment

FIG. 18.—THE LAY-OUT OF A DRESSING TROLLEY

A mackintosh may be needed to protect the bed, particularly if the wound requires irrigating.

Cheatle's Forceps (Instrument forceps). These are
sterilized by boiling and placed in a tall jar containing lysol
1–40 or other suitable disinfectant solution. The container
should be sufficiently deep to keep the blades and the lower
half of the handles submerged in the lotion.

Instruments. The instruments commonly needed for
ward dressings are dissecting forceps (four pairs should be
provided for each dressing), scissors and clip removers.

Instruments taken from the sterilizer should be placed in sterile containers with properly fitting lids.

Lotions. Screw-topped bottles of normal saline and water are sterilized by autoclaving before use and care must be taken to prevent contamination of the contents during use. Once open to the air the fluid is no longer sterile unless special precautions are taken. The closed bottle is preferable for irrigating purposes to the open irrigating can, and for this purpose a length of rubber tubing with a clip and a canula or an irrigating nozzle can be attached to a delivery tube passing through a rubber bung in the neck of the bottle. The whole outfit can be sterilized by autoclaving, or the bottle and its contents may be autoclaved and the fittings sterilized by boiling.

Tulle Gras and Carbonet* Dressings. These are prepared and then sterilized in tins in the autoclave. The strips are removed with sterile forceps when needed.

When setting the dressing trolley articles which will be handled by the dresser or the trolley assistant during the actual dressing of the wound are placed on the top shelf, the bottom shelf is reserved for accessories such as bandages. Bins provided with covers are preferable to open "dirty dressings" bowls or receivers and these should be placed on the floor. A jar containing lysol 1–40 solution, or other suitable disinfectant into which forceps and other instruments can be discarded after use is recommended in place of a kidney dish. Alternatively two paper bags may be attached to the trolley, one for the reception of soiled dressings and one for used instruments.

Since, as has already been stated, hands must always be regarded as contaminated unless covered by sterile gloves, the older method of attempting to sterilize hands by thorough scrubbing has been abandoned in favour of washing the hands in the ordinary way to remove loose particles and surface dirt. The hands are then dried on a clean dry towel. Persons who handle dressing materials and instruments and who carry out the dressing of wounds should endeavour to avoid directly touching any sources of gross contamination, as, for example, soiled dressing material. Sterile material should be handled with forceps. Fingernails should be kept

---

*Carbonet is an open mesh gauze dressing impregnated with water-soluble, non-adherent polyethylene glycol.

short and clean. Hands should be kept in good condition by careful drying after washing and by the use of a hand cream, roughness of the skin and cracks are a danger to the dresser and to the patient.

The Conduct of Dressings

The division of duties between dresser and trolley assistant need to be carefully thought out and understood if good aseptic technique is to be attained. The following rules are based on the Medical Research Council's Memorandum.

Only one wound should be uncovered at a time unless more than one team is working in the ward at once.

Two persons are needed, a dresser who takes off bandages and dressings and attends to the toilet of the wound, and a trolley assistant whose duty it is to look after the trolley and to pass sterile articles to the dresser.

Before commencing dressings both dresser and assistant don masks. These masks need not be sterile but should be boiled and washed after use and placed in a covered receptacle. Sterile gowns and gloves may be needed for some dressings such as burns, which must be regarded as particularly easy to infect. Before the procedure begins the assistant washes and dries her hands.

The dresser turns the bedclothes back gently, removes the bandages and the outer dressing and places these in the bin or in the paper bag provided for this purpose. It is more convenient if the lid of the bin is foot-operated. The dresser then washes and dries her hands. From this stage all work is carried out with sterile forceps, the hands must not come in contact with the wound, the skin around it, sterile dressings lotions or other sterilized material.

The inner dressing is removed with forceps and placed in the destructor bin or in a paper bag.

The assistant opens the sterile dressing packet, taking care to touch only the outside. Any other material required by the dresser is handed to her by the assistant with sterile forceps. The dresser must be careful not to allow her forceps to touch those of the assistant.

The dresser cleans the skin around the wound, changes packing or drains, carries out irrigations or removes stitches as required, using sterile forceps and a strict no-touch technique. Loose particles of skin or stitches that have been removed should be placed on a moistened swab in a large gallipot to avoid the danger of these particles falling into the bed or on to the floor.

The dresser applies the new dressing with forceps and then discards her forceps into the receptacle provided.

The dresser then re-bandages the wound taking care to see that the bandage is correctly and firmly applied so that it will not slip and expose the dressing.

A third helper is useful, if available, to arrange the bedclothes or hold a limb if necessary. After rendering such assistance the nurse should wash and dry her hands before proceeding to other duties.

At the completion of the dressing the assistant removes the used articles and afterwards washes and dries her hands.

The dresser replaces the bedclothes if a third helper is not available, and then washes her hands.

Removal of Sutures and Clips

For the removal of sutures dissecting forceps and sharp-pointed scissors are required.

When removing interrupted sutures the thread is lifted up with the forceps near the knot and is then cut through between the knot and the skin; gentle traction on the stitch before cutting will expose a portion of the stitch which has been under the skin surface. The thread is then pulled with forceps from the other end towards the incision so that the part that has been lying on the surface is not drawn through the tissues. If a continuous suture has been used it is cut through close to the skin at each point where it has beeen taken through the tissues. The cut sections are then removed by gentle traction, taking the same care as in the removal of interrupted stitches to avoid drawing the thread that has been lying on the skin surface through the incision.

For the removal of Michel's clips dissecting forceps and clip-removing forceps are required.

The clip is steadied with the dissecting forceps and then one blade of the clip-removing forceps is passed underneath it.

The clip-removing forceps are then closed nipping the clip in the centre, this will bring its pointed ends free of the incision and it can then be lifted out.

Surgical Fomentation

Wet dressings are seldom used now in surgical treatment but should a fomentation be ordered for a septic wound the procedure indicated below should be followed.

Requirements (in addition to the sterile bowls, dissecting forceps and dressings which will be provided on the dressing trolley):

A piece of lint double the size of the area to be fomented.

A piece of protective material, such as jaconet or oiled silk, large enough to cover the lint when folded double.

Sterile cotton wool of sufficient size to cover the lint and protective and to overlap about one inch all round.

A wringer made of linen towelling or of strong cotton material such as pillow ticking.

Method. The lint is wrapped in the centre of the wringer which is placed in boiling water in a saucepan or small sterilizer with the ends hanging over the sides of the container. The fomentation should be boiled for five minutes. When the dresser is ready the assistant brings the fomentation in the saucepan, or lifts it out of the sterilizer by the dry ends and transfers it to a sterile bowl. She wrings it dry by twisting the ends of the wringer and then unfolds this to expose the lint. The dresser picks up the lint with sterile forceps, shakes it to allow the steam to escape, applies it to the wound, covers the lint with the protective and then with the layer of cotton wool. Since the dressing is usually changed frequently a many-tailed bandage is used to cover it wherever possible in place of a roller bandage.

Dressing a Wound with a Drainage Tube

Rubber tubing is cut to the required length and one or two holes are made in the side of the tube. A safety-pin is inserted through one end to prevent the tube from slipping into the cavity. The surgeon gives definite instructions regarding the removal of the tube. In some cases it is shortened daily before it is finally removed, this is done by easing the tube partly out of the wound, cutting off the required length and inserting a fresh safety-pin. If a tube is to be taken out during the dressing and later reinserted a duplicate tube, or if ordered, a smaller one, should be sterilized in readiness. If the same tube has to be used again it is cleaned and sterilized before being reintroduced. A rubber drainage tube is inserted by grasping it lengthways with sinus forceps and introducing it in the direction of the sinus track. When dressing the wound a piece of gauze is packed lightly round the tube under the safety-pin. If a tube is not to be removed but it is suspected that discharge has collected at the bottom of the wound a sterile rubber catheter may be passed down the tube and the discharge aspirated with a syringe.

Closed Drainage

Instead of allowing the pus from a cavity to escape via an open tube into a dressing, closed drainage may be employed. This method is particularly useful in draining the pleural cavity, the dressing does not require frequent changing as is the case with open drainage and expansion of the lung is assisted as the tube opens below the level of fluid in the

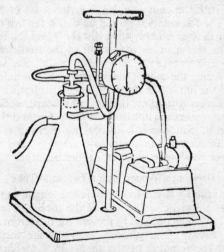

FIG. 19.—SUCTION MOTOR (ELECTRIC) AS USED FOR CAVITY DRAINAGE OR SUCTION OF SOME EMPYEMATA. Note collecting bottle, pressure gauge and release valve and motor.

collecting bottle and, therefore, air is prevented from entering the pleural cavity. The drainage tube is provided with a large rubber flange and must accurately fit the incision in the chest wall. It is connected by a length of rubber tubing to a glass tube passing through the rubber bung of the collecting bottle. The glass tube must be long enough to terminate below the level of the fluid in the bottle. This fluid is usually a disinfectant and deodorant solution such as 30 per cent. chloroxylenol (Dettol). When the bottle is disconnected and removed for emptying and cleaning it is important to clip the rubber tubing first, otherwise air will enter the pleural cavity and the partially expanded lung will collapse. It is also important that the tubing shall not be kinked or obstructed and careful arrangement of the pillows and back rest is necessary in order to support the patient without pressure on the tubing (see page 65). A greater degree of suction can be achieved if necessary by attaching an electric pump or a Sprengel's water pump to a short glass connection passing through the bung of the bottle.

13

Preparation of Patient for Operation and Post-operative Care

CAREFUL pre-operative treatment greatly influences the successful outcome of the operation and the avoidance of post-operative complications. Rest, mental and physical, beforehand is very necessary for the patient who is to undergo a major operation. The nurse's attitude should be one of cheerfulness and confidence but not of indifference to the patient's natural fear and anxiety. The reasons for the various stages of the preparation should be simply explained to the patient before beginning each procedure.

The state of the patient's mouth and teeth should be investigated. The surgeon will decide whether dental treatment is needed. The nurse is responsible for the frequent and thorough cleansing of the patient's mouth as required.

The anæsthetist or the house surgeon will examine the patient's chest. The nurse should report any information that she may have obtained from the patient as, for example, any tendency to bronchitis, a recent cold, an attack of influenza, or the patient's habits with regard to tobacco or alcohol. Breathing exercises may be ordered as a preventive measure against chest complications and these are particularly important in the preparation of the patient for chest and upper abdominal operations.

The bowels should act adequately but violent purgatives tire the intestinal muscle and predispose to post-operative distension. Gentle aperients or enemata are therefore usually ordered, although some surgeons may order castor oil before rectal or perineal operations in order to ensure thorough emptying of the intestinal tract and to inhibit early action of the bowels after operation.

The patient should be encouraged to take sufficient nourishment and the diet should contain a generous allowance of first class protein and vitamins A, B and C. Liberal quantities of fluid and sugar are very valuable, a starved and dehydrated patient is more prone to post-operative complications. If the nature of the patient's disease precludes the intake of sufficient nutriment fluid by mouth intravenous administration of saline-glucose solution is likely to be required.

The general cleanliness of the skin should receive attention, the patient having a daily warm bath in bed or in the bathroom.

The nurse's duties include the testing of the urine, the important abnormalities to be looked for are sugar, acetone, diacetic acid and albumen.

Consent of the patient or responsible relative for the administration of an anæsthetic and for the operation is required and should be obtained in writing. The patient's blood is usually grouped and cross-matched in case blood transfusion is required.

In the case of women patients coloured nail varnish and lipstick should be removed as artificial colour on the lips and nails may mask cyanosis during anæsthesia.

Preparation of the Skin of the Operation Area

A wide area around the operation site is washed and shaved. The skin is then cleaned with ether, surgical spirit or cetrimide. Some surgeons require no further preparation, others will order the skin to be swabbed with an antiseptic ordered by the surgeon, such as chlorhexidine 0·5 per cent. in spirit. Following this the area may be covered with a sterile dressing and a bandage. The preparation for bone operations may begin three days beforehand although some orthopædic surgeons favour only one preparation. The area is cleaned, repainted and covered with a fresh sterile dressing daily, the last application being made immediately before the patient goes to the theatre. In the case of an emergency operation the preparation of the skin is often carried out in the theatre.

Routine Procedure on the Day of Operation

A hypnotic is often ordered to be given on the preceding evening to promote a good night's rest. If a barbiturate drug is used as pre-medication, *e.g.* Nembutal, the first

7+

dose may be given in the evening and the subsequent larger dose about two hours before the operation.

The times at which the various stages of the immediate preparation will be carried out will depend on the time fixed for the operation. The following schedule gives the approximate times when the operation is arranged to take place at 2 p.m. or shortly after.

(1) The early morning specimen of urine is obtained and tested.

(2) A light breakfast of tea and toast is given at 7 a.m. unless there is any contra-indication.

(3) A drink of glucose lemonade or sweetened tea may be given at 10 a.m. unless the anæsthetist's orders are that no fluids should be given after 7 a.m.

(4) At 1 p.m. the patient is dressed in an operation gown and long woollen stockings. The hair is brushed, a woman's hair if long is plaited, tied and covered with a cap or a triangular bandage. Any jewellery, except a wedding ring, is removed and given into the charge of the ward sister. The patient is given a mouth wash, if he is wearing artificial teeth these are now removed and placed in a porringer.

(5) At 1.45 p.m. the patient empties the bladder or is catheterized if this is ordered.

(6) The hypodermic injection of atropine or other pre-operative medication is given at the time ordered, usually three-quarters of an hour before the patient goes to the theatre.

(7) The patient is placed on the theatre trolley. The form of consent for operation, case notes, X-ray films, a vomit bowl, towel, mouth gag, tongue forceps, swabs and swab-holding forceps are all collected and taken to the theatre with the patient.

The nurse accompanies the patient to the anæsthetic room and may remain to assist the anæsthetist, to help wheel the trolley into the theatre and arrange the patient on the operating table. Silence is essential during the induction of the anæsthetic, the nurse should remain quietly at the patient's side and should not speak unless the anæsthetist asks her a question. The ward nurse should be able to answer any questions regarding the patient and his preparation, for example, she should know what pre-medication was given, the time of its administration and the time at which the patient last had any food or fluid.

If a basal anæsthetic such as thiopentone sodium (Pentothal) or pentobarbitone sodium (Nembutal) is given before the patient leaves the ward, he should not be left from the time that the drug is given. Muscular relaxation occurs as the anæsthetic takes effect and the air passage may be obstructed by the tongue falling back. A tray should be ready with a gag, tongue forceps, swab-holding forceps and swabs.

In cases where the operation is a lengthy one, the pre-operative condition of the patient is poor or the loss of blood likely to be considerable, preparations should be made for the transfusion of blood or plasma should this be needed. Oxygen and apparatus for its administration, *e.g.* a B.L.B. mask, should be ready for immediate use. Oxygen with 5 or 7 per cent. carbon dioxide may be required. A hypodermic tray with syringe, needles and stimulants such as nikethamide should be readily available in the event of respiratory or cardiac failure occurring.

When the patient is brought back to the ward sufficient helpers must be available to lift him, with the minimum of disturbance, from the trolley to the bed. The head of the trolley should face the foot of the bed. The top bed-clothes are rolled back and if the bed has been warmed, the electric blanket or hot water bottles are removed, and the warmed blanket is placed next to the patient as he lies on the trolley. Three people will be needed to lift an adult patient; all three should stand in a line at the same side of the trolley. One assistant slides her arms under the patient's head and shoulders; the middle helper takes the heaviest weight of the patient's trunk and if a porter assists the nurses this should be his position, the third assistant puts her arms under the patient's legs. Care should be taken to see that the patient's arm on the far side is not allowed to dangle in such a position that it will be under his body when he is placed in bed. All three persons lift at the same moment, as smoothly as possible, placing the patient gently on his back in the bed. The top bed-clothes are then replaced, the patient's head and shoulders turned to one side and a towel placed under his chin.

The patient must not be left and while he is still deeply

unconscious the nurse who remains at the bedside should
hold the jaw forward by placing her fingers behind the
angle of the jaw in order to keep the tongue forward and
the air-way clear (Fig. 20). If an endotracheal tube or a
rubber airway has been left in it should be removed when
the patient begins to get restless. The pulse rate should be
taken and recorded every quarter-of-an-hour while the

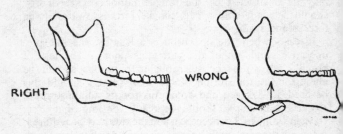

FIG. 20.—RIGHT WAY AND WRONG WAY OF HOLDING THE JAW
OF AN UNCONSCIOUS PATIENT.

patient is unconscious. The strength and volume of the
pulse should be noted, also the colour of the patient, the
rate and depth of the respirations. If the patient is
cyanosed or if his respirations are shallow, oxygen may be
given after making sure that the air-way is not obstructed.

If the patient vomits his head should be turned well to the
side and his mouth mopped out with gauze swabs on sponge
forceps. If his jaw is clenched the gag will be needed and
possibly tongue forceps to pull the tongue forward when the
mouth is opened. The best pattern of tongue forceps have
sharp points which should be inserted into the dorsum of the
tongue on either side of the midline and not through the tip.

The dressing covering the wound should be inspected
frequently; if any blood or serum soaks through, a sterile
dressing should be applied over the bandage without
disturbing the original dressing. Any excessive bleeding
should be reported at once. Should there be a tube from
the operation site that is intended to drain into a receptacle,
this must be attended to as soon as the patient is placed in
bed, the nurse should also make sure that the tube is not
kinked or obstructed in any way. The patient should not
be over-heated by too many blankets and may be more

comfortable if the operation gown and stockings are removed. If hypothermic ("refrigeration") anæsthesia is used the patient is placed in an unwarmed bed and covered only by a sheet. The reason for this is to ensure a gradual rise of the body temperature. A careful watch on the patient's condition and quarter hourly blood pressure readings are necessary.

Except after operations on the stomach and other special cases in which the surgeon may wish a strict régime to be followed, sips of water may usually be given when the patient has recovered from the anæsthetic, swabbing the mouth with a pleasant mouth wash will probably be very acceptable to him, and is particularly necessary if he is not allowed to drink. If vomiting is severe, or if for any reason administration of fluids by mouth is not possible, intravenous fluids are usually given.

The measurement of the urine passed should be kept. If the patient has difficulty in passing urine, and is not helped by such simple measures as sitting upright on a bed-pan containing some warm water and the application of warmth over the lower abdomen, an injection of a parasympathetic stimulant such as carbachol is usually ordered. The patient's bladder must not be allowed to become distended and catheterization may be necessary.

Pain and restlessness should be reported, both will exhaust the patient and may lead to collapse. If morphine or any other sedative has been ordered to be given as and when required, it should be given before the state of exhaustion is reached.

When the patient has recovered from post-operative shock he will usually be nursed in the sitting position. This position encourages free movement of the diaphragm and will help to prevent chest complications. The upright position is also less likely than the recumbent position to favour accumulation of flatus in the intestine. The patient should be encouraged to move his legs freely in bed.

The amount of movement which the individual patient can undertake will, of course, depend on his condition and the type of operation. As a general rule the more the patient moves the better, provided that the operation incision is properly supported where necessary. Movements of the foot and ankle joints will help to prevent stiffness and "dropped foot." Exercise of the quadriceps muscles will assist the venous return and will also help to maintain muscle tone which is so readily lost with inactivity. Deep breathing exercises will help to prevent stagnation at the bases of the lungs and, by increasing the excursion of the diaphragm, will aid the venous return and also promote peristalsis in the intestine helping to prevent distension and constipation.

After most operations early ambulation is the usual procedure, the patient being assisted from his bed to sit in a chair for a short period within forty-eight hours of the operation. The object of this early movement is to avoid the complications of venous thrombosis and pulmonary embolism. The nurse must, however, realize that the fact that the patient leaves his bed does not mean that he is convalescent and he will need a good deal of assistance and encouragement. Everything necessary for his comfort, the chair, blankets and slippers should be prepared and ready before he is moved from his bed and he should be under the observation of the nurse during the whole time that he is out of it.

The time during which the patient will be confined to bed must depend on his general condition and on the nature of the operation. Where firm healing of a plastic operation is essential the patient may be kept in bed for a longer period.

14

Bandaging

Uses of Bandages:

> To fix dressings in position.
> To afford support.
> To arrest hæmorrhage.
> To prevent or reduce swelling.
> To correct deformity.

Types of Bandages:

Roller: 4 to 8 yards long, 1 to 6 inches wide. The parts of the bandage are known as the initial end, the drum and the tail.

Triangular: 1 square yard of material cut diagonally makes two bandages.

Many-tailed: Tails 4 inches wide, the length varies from 42 to 72 inches, width of the back 6 to 8 inches. These measurements are for chest and abdominal bandages.

Jaw or four-tailed: 1 yard long, 4 inches wide, before cutting into tails.

T-bandage: for perineal dressings, 1 yard of 4-inch bandage for the waist band, 1 yard of 6-inch bandage for the perineal strap.

Tubular gauze: For limbs and head bandages.

Material used for Bandages:

Flannel: Strong, warm and gives good support, semi-elastic, but heavy and may be too hot.

Domette: Light, soft and semi-elastic, porous, expensive but washable.

Open-wove cotton: Light and inexpensive, but does not give much support, is washable but the edges fray unless the selvedge edge type is used.

Calico: Harsh and inelastic, but firm; useful for slings and for applying splints.

Crêpe: Comfortable and gives good support, elastic and easy to apply, expensive but washable.

Rules for applying Roller Bandages:

Stand in front of the part to be bandaged.

Pad the axilla or groin when bandaging near these parts.

Start with an oblique turn.

Bandage from below upwards, and from within outwards.

Apply the bandage with firm even pressure throughout.

Cover two-thirds of the previous turn of the bandage leaving one-third uncovered.

The drum of the bandage must be held uppermost.

Reverse on the outside of the limb.

Finish with a spiral turn, turning in the end of the bandage and securing it with a safety-pin arranged with point uppermost.

Points to Remember:

The comfort of the patient is the first consideration except when arresting hæmorrhage or correcting deformity.

Two skin surfaces should not be allowed to lie in contact under the bandage; if this point is not attended to, the skin is liable to become moist and sore.

The position of the part—place the limb in the position in which it can most easily be maintained by the patient without strain.

Neatness and economy of bandage should be considered, but the bandage must fulfil its purpose and must always completely cover the dressing.

Various Patterns used in Roller Bandaging:

Spiral: Used for limbs of uniform dimensions—*e.g.* fingers.

Reversed Spiral: Used for limbs which vary in thickness —*e.g.* forearm.

Figure-of-eight: Used chiefly for joints, but can be adapted for use on any part of the body.

Spica: The name given to a figure-of-eight bandage when applied to joints at right angles to the body—*e.g.* shoulder or thumb.

Ear. Use a 2-inch bandage. Fix by placing the end of the bandage over the ear to be bandaged and taking one-and-a-half turns round the head; then carry the bandage obliquely downwards across the back of the head to cover the lowest portion of the dressing. Continue to carry the bandage forwards and upwards across the horizontal turn and over the side of the head. Repeat the horizontal turn. Repeat these two turns until dressing is covered. Finish with a turn round the head and fasten in front.

Eye. Use a 2-inch "fast edge" bandage. Place the bandage over the ear on the side of the eye to be bandaged. Fix by taking a turn across the brow and around the head. Carry the bandage obliquely down across the back of the head, beneath the ear and up over the eye towards the nose and over the head to the starting point (Fig. 21). Repeat these turns once or twice and finish by pinning the bandage on the forehead over the good eye. The bandage should not obstruct the vision of the good eye.

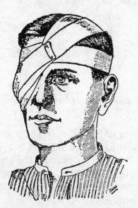

FIG. 21.—EYE BANDAGE.

Double Eye. First and second turns as for single eye. Third turn carry the bandage down over the uncovered eye, beneath the ear and obliquely up the back of the head.

7*

Repeat these turns and finish as before. The crossings should be directly over the nose.

Ascending Spica of Shoulder. Use a 3-inch bandage. Pad the axilla. Fix the bandage with an oblique turn around the arm. Carry the bandage across the back, under the opposite arm and across the chest to the outer side of the arm. Repeat these turns, working up over the shoulder, chest and back until the dressing is covered. Finish over the shoulder in front (Fig. 22).

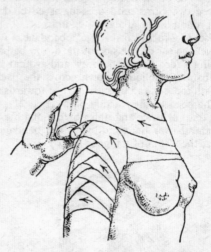

FIG. 22.—ASCENDING SHOULDER SPICA.

Descending Spica of Shoulder. The same turns are made for a descending spica of shoulder as for an ascending one, but the bandage is begun by placing the end on the shoulder and the spicas work downwards over the shoulder, back and chest. The bandage is finished off by taking a circular turn round the arm (Fig. 23).

Breast. Use a 4- or 6-inch bandage. Start beneath the unaffected breast and take one-and-a-half circular turns round the body. The bandage is now beneath the affected breast. Carry the bandage obliquely upwards covering the lowest portion of the dressing, over the shoulder and down the back. Repeat the turn round the body, covering only two-thirds of the previous turn (Fig. 24). Repeat these turns until the breast is sufficiently covered and supported. Finish in front.

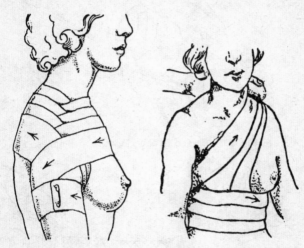

FIG. 23.—DESCENDING SHOULDER SPICA.

FIG. 24.—BREAST BANDAGE.

For all bandages involving the thorax it is important to see that the patient's shoulders are well back when the bandage is applied, otherwise breathing may be impeded.

Flexed Elbow. Use a 2½- or 3-inch bandage. Carry the bandage twice round the centre of the joint. Continue with a figure-of-eight pattern, first above and then below the joint, and covering two-thirds of the previous turn. Finish with a circular turn above the joint (Fig. 25).

Flexed Knee. Use a 3-inch bandage. The method is the same as for a flexed elbow.

Heel. Use a 2-inch bandage. The same pattern of bandage as for an elbow but the first turn of the figure-of-eight is made below the tip of the heel instead of above. Finish around the ankle.

Figure-of-Eight of Arm or Leg. Use a 2- or 2½-inch bandage for the arm and a 3-inch bandage for the leg. Fix

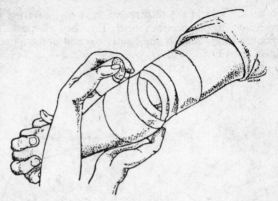

Fig. 25.—Flexed Elbow, Divergent Spica.

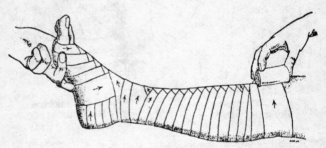

Fig. 26.—Bandage for Foot and Leg, Using Figure-of-Eight and Reversed Turns.

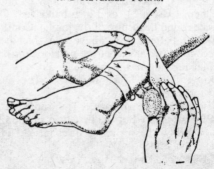

Fig. 27.—Reversed Turn.

by taking one oblique turn round the limb. The pattern is made by carrying the bandage obliquely up, around and down the limb, the loops forming a figure-of-eight. The crossings should be on the outside of the limb in a straight line. Finish with a circular turn. (Fig. 26.)

Reversed Spiral, Arm or Leg. Use a 2½-inch bandage for the arm and a 3-inch bandage for the leg. Fix by taking one oblique turn around the limb. As each successive turn is brought to the front of the limb, reverse the bandage by fixing it with the thumb and turning it obliquely down on itself (Fig. 27). The points formed in this way should be in a straight line on the outside of the limb. Finish with a circular turn.

Hand. Use a 2-inch bandage. Commence by placing the end of the bandage on the inner side of the wrist, then carry the bandage across the back of the hand to the base of the little finger and take a simple spiral turn one-and-a-half times round the knuckles; the bandage is now by the first finger. Start the figure-of-eight turns round the hand and wrist—three or four should be sufficient. Finish with a circular turn round the wrist. The spicas should come in the centre of the back of the hand. If limited movement of the fingers is not allowed a single layer of material should be placed between them.

Fingers. Use a 1-inch bandage. Start on the inner side of the wrist, leaving a free end for tying. Carry the bandage across the back of the hand to the base of the finger to be bandaged; in one elongated turn bring the bandage to the base of the nail and work down the finger in spiral turns. Carry the bandage across the back of the hand and take one turn around the wrist, and either fasten off by tying the ends together or, if another finger is to be bandaged bring the bandage up the finger and repeat these turns. If bandaging all the fingers, start with the little finger.

To cover the tip of the finger: commence as before, but instead of taking a spiral turn up the finger, carry the bandage straight up the outside of the finger over the tip and down the inside of the finger as far as the second joint; hold the bandage there and make a return loop over the tip of the finger once more. Fix the loops with one circular turn, then, commencing at the top of the finger cover in the whole of the finger with spiral turns as before.

Spica for Thumb. Use a 1-inch bandage. Commence from the inner side of the wrist, leaving sufficient to tie. Carry the bandage down between the finger and thumb, then take a single spiral turn around the thumb, followed by a circular turn at the base of the nail. Start the figure-of-eight

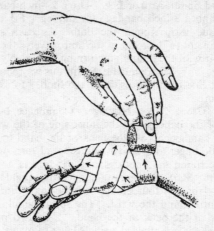

FIG. 28.—SPICA FOR THUMB.

turns by carrying the bandage across the back of the thumb and hand to the wrist, around the wrist and across the ball of the thumb. Repeat these figure-of-eight turns until the thumb is covered (Fig. 28). Finish round the wrist.

Stump. Use a 3- or 4-inch bandage according to the size of the stump. Start by placing the end of the bandage in the centre of the upper side of the stump, then carry the bandage over the centre to the same position on the under side; hold in position with the fingers. Continue to carry the bandage to and fro over the end of the stump until it is completely covered; fix the loops with a circular turn round the stump. Continue up the stump with a figure-of-eight bandage until the dressing is covered. The spica of the bandage should be on the upper side of the stump. This bandage is used to retain the dressing for a few days following amputation. Later, a special crêpe bandage may be applied to exert pressure and prevent œdema of the stump.

Ascending Spica of Hip. Use a 4- or 6-inch bandage. Pad the groin. Fix the bandage with one oblique turn around the thigh. Carry the bandage obliquely upwards to the outside of the hip, around the back and down across the pelvis to the outside of the thigh. Continue these two turns, the spica ascending on the front and outside of the thigh. Finish on the trunk in front.

Descending Spica of Hip. Apply in the same way as an ascending spica, but start with a figure-of-eight turn around

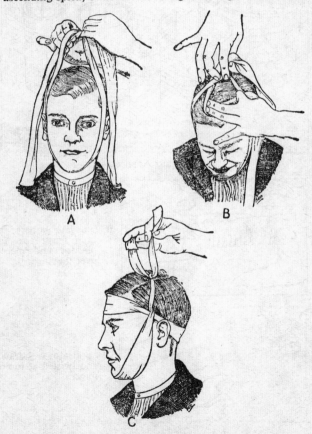

A   B

C

FIG. 29.—THE BARREL BANDAGE.

the trunk and thigh. The spica works downwards instead
of upwards and the bandage is finished with a circular turn
round the thigh.

Ankle. Use a 2-inch bandage. Start with an oblique

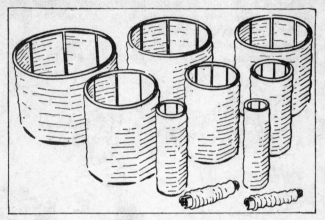

A, Tubegauz Applicators.

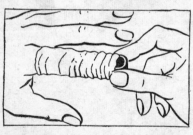

B, Tubegauz gathered on
to a finger size ap-
plicator and placed
over the finger.

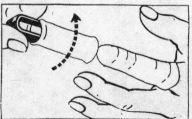

C, Applicator withdrawn
and twisted at top of
finger.

FIG. 30.—"TUBEGAUZ" BANDAGES.

turn round the instep and proceed with figure-of-eight turns around the instep and ankle, working upwards with the spica on the front of the foot and ankle until sufficient support is obtained. Finish with a circular turn around the ankle.

The "Barrel" Bandage for supporting a Fractured Jaw. A strip of bandage about 4 feet long and 2 inches wide is required. This is placed under the chin and tied in a single knot on the top of the head (Fig. 29A). The knot is then loosened and spread out so that one loop passes round the back of the head and the other round the forehead (Fig. 29B). The tails of the bandage are then tied on the top of the head (Fig. 29C).

"Tubegauz" Bandages

Tubular gauze bandages have recently found favour as a comfortable, neat and efficient method of retaining dressings in position. The gauze is made in various dimensions suitable for many purposes. For bandaging limbs wire cage applicators on which the gauze is stretched are used. (Fig. 30.) The applicator is passed over the part to be bandaged and then withdrawn leaving a layer of gauze covering the area. This procedure is repeated to give as many layers as are necessary covering the part.

It is claimed that a great degree of control over the tension of the bandage is possible with this method and also that the bandage will retain its position better than the usual roller bandage. Many casualty departments find that "Tubegauz" is particularly useful for finger dressings and that the light, neat bandage is greatly appreciated by patients. "Tubegauz" also makes a satisfactory and comfortable head bandage.

Triangular Bandages

SLINGS

Large Arm Sling (used to support the forearm). Stand in front of the patient. Spread the bandage over the chest, with one end going over the shoulder on the uninjured side, and the other hanging over the abdomen; the point should be beneath the elbow. Place the forearm slightly raised over the middle of the sling; bring the lower end up and tie on the injured shoulder to the other end with a reef knot. Tuck in the ends. Bring the point round to the front of the elbow, fold in neatly and pin (Fig. 31A).

Narrow Arm Sling (used to support the wrist). Make a broad fold bandage by bringing the point to the base and folding in two. Place one end over the shoulder on un-injured side. Place the wrist on the centre of the broad fold and bring the lower end up to the injured shoulder. Join ends with a reef knot (Fig. 31B).

St. John Sling (used when the shoulder is injured and to give support to a fractured clavicle). Place the injured arm across the chest so that the fingers almost touch the

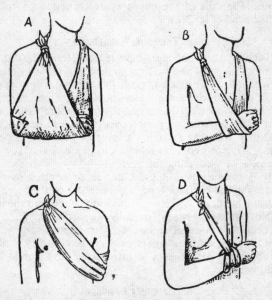

FIG. 31.—ARM SLINGS.
A, large arm sling; B, narrow arm sling; C, St. John sling; D, clove-hitch as sling.

opposite shoulder. Place one end of the bandage on the uninjured shoulder so that the point comes well beyond the elbow. Tuck the upper half of the base of the bandage well beneath the forearm and elbow. Carry the lower end across the back and tie the ends on the uninjured shoulder. Tuck the point in between the forearm and the sling. Carry the fold thus made around the outside of the arm and pin firmly to the bandage going up the back (Fig. 31c).

Clove-hitch. With hands 8 inches apart and palms uppermost, hold the bandage between the fingers and thumb of either hand. Turn the palms downwards, at the same time throwing the tail in the right hand over the bar of the bandage. Turn the right palm upwards with the loop around the fingers and slip the lower part of the loop from the left hand on to the right hand without altering its position. The two loops are then on the right hand and the clove hitch is completed (Fig. 31D).

OTHER USES

Scalp. Fold a hem of about $1\frac{1}{2}$ inches along the base of the bandage. Stand behind the patient. Place the bandage over the head with the centre of the base on the forehead, the hem outwards and the point resting on the nape of the neck. Bring the ends around the head, crossing at the back and tying over the centre of the forehead. Draw the point of the bandage down as far as possible, then turn it up and pin it to the bandage on top of the head.

Forehead, Eye and Side of Head. Make a narrow fold by bringing the point to the base and folding in three. Place the centre of the bandage over the dressing, carry the ends around the head and tie.

Chest. Place the centre of the bandage on the dressing, with the point over the shoulder on the injured side. Carry the ends around the waist, leaving one end longer than the

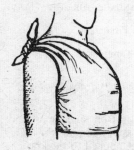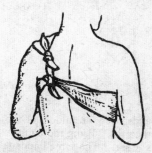

FIG. 32.—TRIANGULAR BANDAGE FOR THE CHEST.
A, front view; B, bandage secured at the back.

other. Draw the point over the shoulder and tie to this end (Fig. 32).

Back. The back is bandaged in the same way, beginning at the back and knotting the bandage in front.

Shoulder. Two bandages are required. Fold a hem at the base of one bandage and place the centre of the bandage on the shoulder with the point running up the side of the neck. Carry the ends around the middle of the arm and tie on the outer side. Place the arm on the injured side in a broad fold sling, tying the knot over the point of the bandage. Draw down the point over the knot and pin.

Elbow. Fold a hem along the base of the bandage. Place the point of the bandage on the back of the arm and the middle of the base on the back of the forearm. Cross the

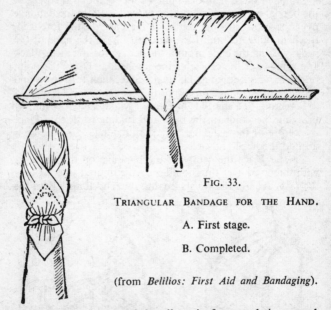

Fig. 33.

Triangular Bandage for the Hand.

A. First stage.

B. Completed.

(from *Belilios: First Aid and Bandaging*).

ends over the middle of the elbow in front and tie around the arm. Bring the point over the knot and pin.

Knee. The same bandage may be applied to the knee.

Hand. Fold a hem along the base of the bandage. Place the wrist on the centre of the base, palm downwards and fingers towards the point. Bring the point over the hand to the wrist, pass the ends around the wrist, or cross and tie. Pull the point over the knot and pin to bandage (Fig. 33).

Hip. Two bandages are required. Tie a narrow fold bandage around the body just above the iliac crests, with

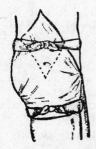

FIG. 34.—TRIANGULAR BANDAGE FOR THE HIP.

the knot on the injured side. Pass the point of the second bandage underneath the knot of the first and fold over. Make a hem along the base of the bandage, pass ends round the thigh and tie. Fasten the point of the bandage down with a safety pin (Fig. 34).

Foot. Place the foot on the centre of the bandage, toes towards the point. Bring the point over the instep. Cross the ends over the instep, carry round the ankle and tie. Pull the point over the knot and pin it.

15

Splints: Plaster of Paris Application: Traction

Splints

SPLINTS may be applied to immobilize a part, to correct or prevent a deformity, or for protection.

Various types of wooden and metal splints are made for splinting different parts of the body.

Splints used on the Lower Extremity

Thomas's Knee Splint (Fig. 35). This splint is used with traction in the treatment of a fractured femur. A modification of the Thomas's splint is the walking caliper, frequently ordered for a patient with a fractured femur when he is allowed up. The lower end of the splint fits into sockets made in the heel of the boot; the ring of the splint takes some of the body weight when the patient walks.

Böhler's Walking Splint (Fig. 36) is incorporated in a plaster splint for the treatment of fractures of the lower part of the leg.

Braun's Cradle Splint (Fig. 37) is used with extension in the treatment of fractures of the lower limb.

Cramer's Wire Splint (Fig. 38) is a malleable "universal" type of splinting which can be cut to the required length and adapted to a variety of purposes.

Splints used on the Upper Extremity

"Cock-up" Splint (Fig. 39). This is a malleable metal splint used to maintain the wrist and hand in the position of extension.

"Aeroplane" Splint (Fig. 40). This splint supports the arm in a position of abduction in the treatment of fractures of the upper end of the humerus.

Gooch's corrugated wood splinting, which may be cut to any size required, may be used as a "first-aid" support

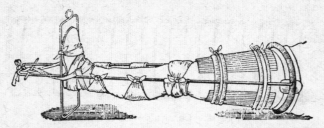

FIG. 35.—THOMAS'S KNEE SPLINT AS APPLIED FOR FIRST AID
TREATMENT OF A FRACTURED FEMUR.

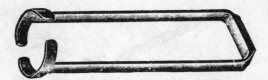

FIG. 36.—BÖHLER'S WALKING SPLINT.

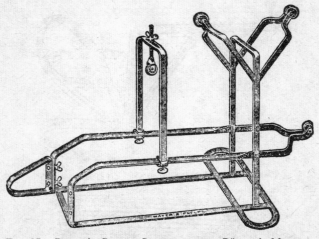

FIG. 37.—BRAUN'S CRADLE SPLINT, USED IN BÖHLER'S METHOD
OF EXTENSION FOR THE LOWER LIMB.

The splint illustrated has been slightly modified from the
original; the upper end has been shortened on one side in order
that the metal frame shall not press uncomfortably tightly in
the groin.

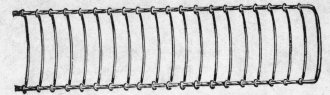

FIG. 38.—CRAMER'S WIRE SPLINT.

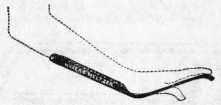

FIG. 39.—METAL "COCK-UP" SPLINT.

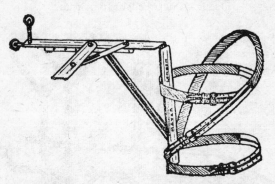

FIG. 40.—"AEROPLANE" SPLINT.

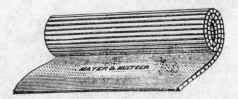

FIG. 41.—GOOCH'S SPLINTING.

for a fracture. It is sometimes used to prevent movement, for which purpose it may be applied to a child's arms to prevent interference with dressings.

Points which should receive Attention in the Application of a Splint.

(1) The limb should be washed and, if adhesive plaster is to be used, the skin may require to be shaved before this is applied.

(2) The splint should be adequately padded, especially over bony prominences.

(3) The splint should be comfortable.

(4) The splint should achieve its object.

Padding Splints. In cases where a splint is to be applied only as a temporary measure it may be padded with non-absorbent wool fixed by a bandage. When the splint is likely to be worn for some time, a more satisfactory padding is applied as described below.

Requirements:
  Calico.
  Wool.
  Good quality tow, hair is sometimes used for special
    splints.
  Linen thread.
  Scissors.
  Sewing cotton and needles.

Method. Cut a piece of calico three times the width of the splint to be padded and at least 6 inches longer.

Cut a piece of wool slightly wider and longer than the splint.

Tease sufficient tow to make a thick springy pad, placing the tow on the wool.

Cover the pad with calico, stitch the pad along its length, but leave the ends open.

Place the pad on the side of the splint which will be next to the patient, with the seam of the pad against the splint.

With the linen thread attach the pad to the splint, taking stitches backwards and forwards across the back of the splint, pulling the thread as tightly as possible. Begin 3 inches from the end and finish off 3 inches from the other end.

At each end make a bar by taking several horizontal stitches across the back of the splint.

Turn in the open ends of the calico and attach them to the cross bars at either end with the splint stitch.

Buttonhole stitch along the cross bar to keep the stitches in place.

Plaster of Paris Splints

Plaster of Paris splints are in general use in the treatment of injuries. Since the splint is made individually for each patient, it is more efficient and more comfortable than most wooden or metal ones.

The following requirements are usually sufficient for the making of the plaster splint although some surgeons may have additions to make to this list for special plasters:

Pails filled with tepid water for soaking the bandages.

Mackintoshes.

Gypsona plaster bandages of the required widths.

Plaster knives.

Ordinary round-ended scissors and plaster scissors such as Böhler's scissors.

Plaster saw.

Plaster shears will be needed if a plaster has to be removed before the application of a fresh one.

Tape measure.

Blue pencil.

Dusting powder may be used for the patient's skin or, if the plaster is being applied without any padding, the skin may be oiled with olive oil.

A light coating of petroleum jelly may be applied to the inside surface of pails in which bandages are soaked in order to facilitate the subsequent removal of hardened plaster. This is not necessary if plastic pails are used.

A suitable table top or a board is needed for the making of plaster slabs.

Tubular stockinet may be used to cover the limb under the plaster or, in the case of the trunk, a stockinet vest.

Dressmaker's wadding, thick felt or sorbo rubber may be used as padding over bony prominences.

Rolls of "orthopædic" or tailor's wool.

Crêpe bandages.

Open wove cotton bandages.

In the theatre the surgeon is usually already dressed in gloves, a rubber apron and theatre boots; otherwise these should be provided. Canvas over-boots may be used in place of rubber ones.

The pail or bowl provided for soaking the bandages should be deep enough to contain sufficient water completely to submerge the bandages. The bandages are placed in water one at a time and left until all the air has bubbled out of the bandage and the water has soaked through to the centre. When the bubbling has ceased the bandage is removed from the water holding it by both ends and gently squeezed towards the centre so that surplus water is removed but the plaster is not squeezed out.

Plaster Bandages. If Gypsona bandages are not available plaster bandages may be prepared by the following method.

For the foundation of the bandages either butter muslin, which is a thin soft material, or book muslin, which is also thin but stiff, is used. The material is torn into lengths of from one to six yards and varying widths of which four, six and seven inches are the most generally useful. Narrow bandages of one or two inches are usually made one or two yards in length, the wider bandages, six, seven or eight inches, are made in lengths of five or six yards.

The strips of material are folded and loose threads removed. The dry plaster is then rubbed into the material as evenly as possible, using the flat part of the palm of the hand. A short strip of muslin is unfolded at a time and loosely rolled as the plaster is rubbed into the mesh. It is convenient to run a red thread through the free end of the finished bandage so that the end may be easily found after the bandage has been soaked. Until sufficient experience has been gained in rolling plaster bandages some difficulty may be found in gauging the right amount of dry plaster to impregnate the muslin properly so that it is not, on the one hand, so full of plaster that the centre of the bandage remains dry when it is immersed in water and, on the other hand, so deficient in plaster as to be finally little more than a piece of wet muslin. Another common mistake is to roll the bandages so tightly that the water cannot soak completely through and a considerable portion of the bandage is wasted. A fine quality quick-setting plaster should be used. If it has not been stored in airtight tins it may be lumpy, and in this case should be sieved before use. The finished bandages should also be stored in airtight tins and may with advantage be dried out in a warm oven before being put away.

The Applications of a Plaster Splint. The nurse will often have to assist in the application of the splint, and in some circumstances may be entrusted with the carrying out of the entire procedure. Plaster bandages should be applied evenly but not tightly and no reverses should be made. The bandage should be folded to bring about a change in the direction of the turn. Plaster sets quickly and the moulding of the casing to the limb should be done during the application of the bandages. "Moulding" means pressing the plaster into the natural hollow contours of the part to which it is applied so that it fits the part accurately and pressure on bony prominences is as far as possible avoided. Reinforcement of the splint may be carried out by strips of plaster bandage applied up and down the length of the limb and secured by further circular turns. Metal strips or pieces of Cramer's wire splinting are sometimes incorporated in a plaster splint. The finished splint should not be subjected to pressure, as for example by letting the heel of a leg plaster rest on the table, until it has set; this usually takes about five minutes. The limb should be supported on the flat of the hand in order to avoid making indentations in the plaster. Thorough drying of the plaster takes several hours, the time depending on the size and thickness of the plaster.

Plaster slabs are often used for limbs and have the advantages of being quick and simple to make, supplying a well-fitting splint which can be removed for any necessary treatment. The length is marked on a board or table and wet plaster bandages are folded lengthways up and down the marked area on the board until the requisite thickness is obtained. The slab of bandage is applied to the limb, moulded and then removed and trimmed. The splint is kept in place by a roller bandage.

Plaster shells may be used in the treatment of disease or injury of the spine. These are made by immersing long strips of muslin eight folds thick in thin plaster cream. The strips are applied and moulded on the patient's body usually directly onto the skin which may be previously oiled. One pound of dry plaster mixed with one pint of water makes a cream of the right consistency. The shell is removed for drying, trimmed and lined with wool or gamgee tissue before use.

Following the application of a plaster the limb should be elevated and the bedclothes arranged over a cradle so as to allow free circulation of air to dry the plaster. The extremities should be inspected hourly for signs of interference with the circulation. If sufficient pressure is applied to the skin to blanch it the colour should return in a few seconds when the pressure is removed. If the skin remains white for any appreciable time this indicates inadequate circulation; blueness and coldness of the extremities are also danger signs. These signs should be reported at once as the plaster will probably have to be cut away or split and opened. After forty-eight hours, routine morning and evening inspection is in most cases sufficient. A sore may develop under the plaster and any complaint of pain at a definite point or a burning sensation should be reported at once, the area subjected to pressure soon becomes anæsthetic and the fact that the pain has disappeared does not mean that the danger of a pressure sore has passed. If a sore forms, the site may be indicated by the presence of a discharge on the surface of the plaster, the presence of a sore may also be detected by the unpleasant smell which develops when discharge is pent up under the splint. When a leg plaster is carried up to the groin special care is needed to prevent soiling. A piece of jaconet or plastic material may be required for protection of the plaster when the patient uses a bed-pan.

To remove a Plaster. The plaster should be removed in a plaster room or a ward annexe otherwise infected loose particles are liable to be scattered and will add to the bacterial content of the air in the ward. The plaster should be moistened during the removal to reduce scattering of dry plaster.

A small light plaster can usually be removed by cutting through it with a knife. Great care must be taken to avoid cutting the patient's skin when removing an unpadded plaster, and in this case a pair of plaster scissors is to be preferred. Plaster shears or an electric saw will be required for cutting through a thick plaster.

After removal the plaster cast should be placed in a covered bin. The knives, scissors and shears should be boiled after use.

Plastic Splints

Light-weight splints made of plastics or resins are useful for infants and in cases where the splint is worn for a considerable time as, for example, in the treatment of a fracture of the scaphoid bone in the wrist. Some of these materials are inflammable and some may cause irritation of the skin.

The Application of Traction

Traction or extension is applied to a limb in order to exert a steady pull. This may be needed to prevent over-riding of the fragments of a fracture or to prevent pain and contractures in the treatment of joint conditions, such as rheumatoid arthritis or tuberculous joints.

Traction may be carried out by the continuous pull of weights, or by fixed traction when the pull is maintained by fixation to the end of the splint. The traction may be applied to the skin of the limb, skin traction, or to the bone, skeletal traction. The latter is obtained by a pin or wire inserted through the bone below the fracture. In the case of a fracture of the lower limb skeletal traction is usually applied at one of three sites, the lower end of the femur just above the condyles, the tubercle of the tibia or the os calcis. For skin traction strips of adhesive material, such as Elastoplast extension strapping, are applied to the skin of the limb, or strips of gauze may be stuck to the skin with Sinclair's glue or Mastisol.

Preparation for Application of Extension:

(1) *The bed* (see also p. 64):

Fracture boards will be needed to prevent sagging of the mattress.

Blocks are often required for raising the foot of the bed.

A Balkan beam, Hoskins's overhead beam or some other type of frame with pulleys, will be needed unless a Braun's cradle splint is to be used.

(2) *The Splint.* If a Thomas's splint is used it must be the right size for the patient, the ring should fit comfortably in the groin resting against the ischial tuberosity at the back and the splint should be long enough to project about six to eight inches beyond the sole of the foot. A flexion bar is usually attached to the splint to allow flexion of the knee joint.

A Hodgen's splint is sometimes used for fractures of the shaft of the femur. This splint is somewhat similar to the Thomas's knee splint, but at the upper end in place of the padded ring of the Thomas's splint there is an anterior wire hoop which is not padded. Unlike the Thomas's splint, it cannot be used for either right or left leg and care must be taken to provide the correct splint for the limb to be treated. Braun's splint is used in the Böhler method of treating fractures of the lower limb. High blocks are required for the foot of the bed and the splint needs to be firmly lashed to the foot of the bed. If the bed is not on a sufficiently inclined plane from the foot towards the head, and if the splint is not firmly anchored to the foot of the bedstead it may press uncomfortably in the patient's groin.

Whichever type of splint is used, flannel slings or bandages will be needed to support the limb. The slings are attached by large spring paper-clips or by safety-pins to one side of the splint. When it has been applied to the limb each sling is adjusted separately and secured. The upper and lower edges of each sling should overlap the slings above and below, if a gap is left the edges of the sling may press into the soft tissues of the limb.

Support for the foot in order to maintain it in a position of dorsiflexion may be supplied in several ways, *e.g.* a foot support attached to the splint, or a cord and a weight attached to a wooden spreader fixed to the sole of a slipper worn on the foot of the fractured limb, the pull of the weight will be towards the head.

(3) *Requirements for Skin Traction:*

Adhesive strapping, "orthopædic" strapping, is the most suitable type as it will not stretch lengthways although it will stretch in width allowing it accurately to fit the limb.

A wooden spreader with a hole in the centre for the cord carrying the weight. The spreader separates the two lengths of strapping along the limb and prevents pressure on the prominences of the malleoli at the ankle. The strapping may enclose the spreader or may be fastened to it by webbing and buckles.

Extension cord and pulleys.

Padding for bony prominences such as the condyles of

the tibia head of the fibula and the malleoli. Folds
of flannel, pieces of felt or wool may be used.

Crêpe, domette or woven edge cotton bandages, 3, 3½
and 4 inches wide.

Safety-pins.

Tape measure.

Scissors.

Weights.

Requisites for shaving the limb should be provided,
although some surgeons prefer to apply the strapping
to the unshaved skin.

Method of Applying the Adhesive Strapping to the Skin.
The width of the strapping used is from 3 to 5 inches,
according to the size of the limb. It may be wider at the
upper end and narrowed by being folded in at the distal
end. The length of the two strips to be applied to the outer
and inner aspects of the limb will be measured from the
level on the limb indicated by the surgeon to about 3 inches
below the sole of the foot. The last 8 inches are narrowed
by cutting or turning in, and covered on the adhesive side
with an 8-inch strip of plaster of the same width in order
to provide a non-sticky surface in contact with the ankle.
The edges of the long strips are snipped at intervals to
allow the strapping to fit the limb without wrinkling. An
alternative method is to cut the strapping lengthways in
three narrow strips as far as the lower 8 or 10 inches, the
three strips can be separated and, when applied to the skin,
will lie more smoothly than one wide piece. The double
thickness of strapping at the lower end is attached to the
buckles of the stirrup or spreader. If the spreader is to be
enclosed in the strapping then two pieces are cut, one
double the length of the single strips referred to above, and
a shorter strip about 10 inches long. The spreader is
placed in the centre of the long strip against the adhesive
surface. The second strip is placed, also adhesive surface
down, over the middle section of the long strip so that both
strips are enclosing the spreader and a non-sticky surface
is provided wherever the strapping may come in contact
with the ankle. A hole is made in the strapping to correspond with the hole in the centre of the spreader. A crêpe
or woven cotton bandage is applied over the strapping

beginning at a point well above the prominence of the malleoli. A system of pulleys, cords and balancing weights is usually arranged to allow the patient to adjust his position. He is encouraged to exercise the muscles and joints by movement which can be carried out safely as the traction through the long axis of the fractured bone is constant.

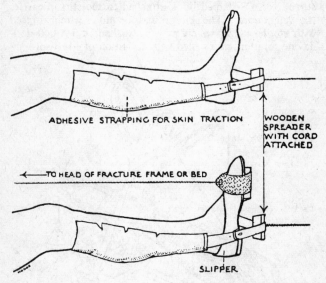

ADHESIVE STRAPPING FOR SKIN TRACTION

WOODEN SPREADER WITH CORD ATTACHED

←—TO HEAD OF FRACTURE FRAME OR BED

SLIPPER

FIG. 42.—APPLICATION OF ADHESIVE STRAPPING FOR SKIN TRACTION AND METHOD OF APPLYING SLIPPER AND CORD FOR THE PREVENTION OF "FOOT-DROP."

Vertical Extension with Skin Traction. This method is used in the treatment of fractures of the femur in young children under the age of six. Both the fractured and the sound limb are suspended vertically to a beam across the cot. The buttocks are lifted clear of the bed and the child's body acts as the counter-weight. In this position the child is easily attended to and the soiling of strappings or bandages is avoided.

Skeletal Traction. The insertion of the pin or wire is carried out in the theatre. Steinmann's pin, which has a sharp point at one end and a nail head at the other, is

8+

hammered through the bone and the ends of the pin are held in a metal stirrup. Böhler's rotating stirrup is commonly used. The cord carrying the weight is attached to the ring of the stirrup.

Kirschner's wire is inserted through the bone by means of a drill and the ends of the wire are held in a horseshoe metal stirrup. An S-shaped hook attached to the stirrup carries the weight cord. The skin around the pin or wire is dressed with sterile gauze, which may be soaked in 1–1,000 acriflavine solution, and sealed with collodion or Mastisol.

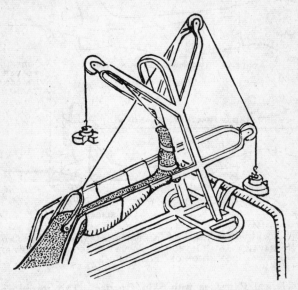

FIG. 43.—SKELETAL TRACTION USED WITH A BRAUN'S SPLINT IN THE TREATMENT OF A FRACTURED FEMUR.

Weight. The amount of weight used for traction will depend on the fracture and on the weight and muscular development of the patient. An average amount is 2 pounds for every stone of body weight, although a greater weight may be applied for the first few days, in order to overcome the powerful contraction of the muscles, and later reduced.

Following the application of an extension the nurse should attend to the following points:

  (i) The weight must exert continuous pull. At no time should the weight be lifted or allowed to rest on the bed.

 (ii) The cord must run freely over the pulley.

(iii) The foot must be supported and kept warm.

 (iv) Where a Thomas's or Hodgen's splint is used the limb and the splint must swing clear of the bed when the patient moves the splint, and the limb should be so balanced that they remain in position.

  (v) When skin traction has been used the extension should be frequently inspected to make sure that the adhesive strapping has not slipped or wrinkled (in which case it is likely to cause a sore) or that it has not broken.

 (vi) Pressure areas, such as the medial and lateral malleoli and the head of the fibula, should be well protected by padding.

16

Observation of Vomit, Sputum, Urine and Stools: Urine Testing: Collection of Specimens for Laboratory Examination

Observation of Vomit

VOMITING is a muscular action which results in the contents of the stomach being ejected through the mouth. The nerve centre from which the muscles concerned receive their messages is in the medulla of the brain, and this vomiting centre may be stimulated in various ways.

Peripheral Stimulation. Afferent messages reach the centre from outside the brain:—

(1) as a result of irritation in the stomach, either due to some abnormal condition of the organ or to some irritating quality in the stomach contents;

(2) as a result of severe pain, especially of the "colic" type;

(3) as a result of an abnormal condition in the abdomen, *e.g.* intestinal obstruction;

(4) by a variety of stimuli, which will vary in individuals, as, for example, an unpleasant sight or smell, or the disturbance produced by the movement of a boat, aeroplane or train.

Central Stimulation. Nerve cells in the brain are directly stimulated by:

(1) Any condition in which the intracranial pressure is increased—*e.g.* cerebral tumour/cerebral abscess, meningitis, concussion.

(2) Poisons circulating in the blood, *e.g.* bacterial toxins, drugs, products of abnormal metabolism, or excess of waste products retained in the blood.

Note should be taken of the following points with regard to vomiting:

(1) Whether preceded by complaint of nausea or by retching.
(2) Whether the vomiting occurs at any particular time of the day, and if it is related to the taking of food.
(3) Whether it is associated with any particular article in the diet.
(4) Whether it is preceded by or accompanied by pain.
(5) Whether pain is relieved by vomiting.
(6) Whether the vomiting is forcible in character— "projectile vomiting."
(7) Whether the vomiting is regurgitant in character.

The material vomited should be saved for inspection and note made of the quantity of the vomit and the number of times vomiting occurs in twenty-four hours. Commonly the vomit consists of food or liquid recently ingested and mixed with mucus.

Bilious or green vomit is due to the presence of bile and is seen when the vomiting continues after the stomach has been emptied of food.

Dark-brown foul-smelling fluid is vomited in intestinal obstruction after preliminary vomiting of food and bile, it is often referred to as "fæcal vomiting."

Blood may be vomited as a result of damage to the stomach wall by corrosive poisons, by ulcers or new growths, or from rupture of œsophageal veins. Blood may also be vomited if it has reached the stomach from the nose, nasopharynx or pharynx. The vomiting of blood is referred to as hæmatemesis.

Blood which has been in the stomach for a time is changed by the gastric juice and when vomited is a brown colour and is compared in appearance to coffee grounds.

Very profuse vomiting occurs in acute dilatation of the stomach, which may be a post-operative complication of abdominal operations, and in hypertrophy of the stomach resulting from a narrowing of the opening into the duodenum (pyloric stenosis).

Hyperemesis is a term applied to persistent vomiting, and is usually used to describe the condition of exaggeration of the common morning sickness of pregnancy.

Observation of Sputum

Sputum is material which is expelled from the respiratory

passages. Such material should be received into a sputum container, and, especially in infectious lung conditions such as tuberculosis, the use of handkerchiefs for the reception of sputum should be forbidden. The quantity and type of sputum should be noted, and also whether the patient expectorates it easily or if it is tenacious.

(For instructions in dealing with sputum and cleaning sputum mugs see p. 23, for collection of specimens of sputum see p. 200.)

Mucoid Sputum. This is clear mucus, tenacious in character, usually seen in the early stages of inflammatory conditions such as pneumonia or bronchitis. It is similar in appearance to the secretion from the nasal passage in the early stage of an ordinary cold.

Mucopurulent Sputum. A mixture of pus and mucus seen in the resolving stage of an acute inflammatory condition, and also in chronic infections such as tuberculosis and chronic bronchitis. In some cases it may originate in the nose or nasal sinuses.

Purulent sputum consists of pus coughed up from dilated bronchioles (bronchiectasis), or from the rupture into a bronchus of a lung abscess or of an abscess in an adjacent structure.

Blood-stained Sputum. Rusty-coloured sputum is often seen in pneumonia, the blood has altered in colour and is mixed with the mucoid material. Streaks of bright red blood in the sputum may come from the gums or from congested mucous membrane anywhere in the respiratory tract. If the blood originates in the lung the sputum will be coloured for several days.

Hæmoptysis is the term used to describe the coughing up of blood in any quantity. The blood is bright red and frothy. Hæmoptysis most commonly occurs in pulmonary tuberculosis, bronchiectasis and carcinoma of the bronchus. It may also be due to a pulmonary infarct or to the rupture of an aortic aneurysm.

Fœtid Sputum. Extremely offensive material is expectorated in gangrene of the lung, advanced bronchiectasis and tuberculosis with cavity formation. Such sputum, if allowed to stand in a specimen glass, will separate into three layers. The upper layer is frothy, the middle layer turbid and the bottom layer shows a deposit of pus and shreds of tissue.

Abundant frothy sputum is characteristic of acute œdema of the lung, and may occur in cases of high blood pressure, cardiac or renal disease, asthma, or following inhalation of irritating fumes such as phosgene or chlorine gas.

Observation of Urine

Normal urine is a clear amber fluid with a characteristic odour, having a slightly acid reaction, and a specific gravity of 1,004 to 1,025. The specific gravity of urine is weight of 1 litre of urine compared with the weight of 1 litre of water which is 1,000 grammes. The weight of 1 litre of urine normally varies from 1,004 grammes when the urine is diluted as a result of a high fluid intake, to 1,025 grammes or higher when the urine is concentrated as the result of restricted fluid intake or excessive fluid loss by sweating.

The average amount passed daily is about 1,500 mils (52 oz.). Normal urine consists of water, urea and other nitrogenous waste, chlorides, urates, phosphates and a pigment of uncertain origin named urochrome.

The amount of water excreted varies according to the fluid intake and the needs of the body, the amount of salts excreted will also be a variable quantity but the amount of urea excreted in health on a normal diet is constant.

The urine passed in the early morning is usually required for testing, but in all emergency cases a specimen of urine should be obtained as soon as possible. The specimen should be put up in a clean glass, covered and labelled with the patient's name, the date, and the time at which the urine was passed.

To collect a Specimen from an Infant. *Male.*—A test tube may be placed over the penis and strapped to the anterior abdominal wall.

Female.—A bowl may be placed under the perineum and the anus packed off with wool.

To collect a Twenty-four Hour Specimen of Urine—*e.g.* from 8 a.m. to 8 a.m.:

At 8 a.m. the patient passes urine and this urine is discarded. Each time after this that urine is passed the whole amount is emptied into a large jar or jug kept for the purpose and clearly labelled with the date, ward and patient's name. At 8 a.m. the next morning the patient passes urine and this amount is added to that already in the jar. The specimen is now complete and should be measured. The entire contents of the jar may be required, or in some cases, after measurement of the amount, two specimens are put up for the laboratory. If the urine is to be examined for tubercle bacilli the sediment from the bottom of the jar will be required.

It is important that the twenty-four hour specimen should be complete, and for female patients two bedpans will be required when the bowels are opened.

Toluol or chloroform may be used as preservative, a few drops are added with every fresh addition of urine to the jar.

Alteration in the colour of urine is usually due to concentration, but may be due to:

(1) Blood: when the urine may be coloured red or the blood may give it a smoky, dark appearance.

(2) Bile: when the urine varies from brown to a dark green or almost black colour.

(3) Certain drugs colour the urine—*e.g.* santonin, which gives an orange colour.

(4) Dyes excreted in the urine will alter the colour, *e.g.* a blue colour is shown after the injection of indigo-carmine.

Odour. (1) An ammoniacal smell. This is usually due to decomposition; on standing, the urea is converted by bacterial action into carbonate of ammonia. In cystitis the urine may be alkaline when freshly passed, and the odour of ammonia may be noticed.

(2) Acetone gives a sweetish odour which has been compared with that of new-mown hay.

(3) Infection with *Bacterium coli* gives a fishy smell.

Reaction. Normal urine is slightly acid.

The acidity or alkalinity of urine may be tested with red and blue litmus paper. Acid urine turns blue litmus red, alkaline urine turns red litmus blue. More accurate determination of the pH (the formula for expressing acidity or alkalinity of nearly neutral solutions) is made in the laboratory. Urine may be alkaline in cases of cystitis, if the specimen tested is stale, if the patient is on a vegetarian or very low protein diet, or if the patient is taking alkalis in any quantity by mouth.

N.B.—If the urine is alkaline it should be acidified before carrying out chemical tests.

Specific Gravity. This is recorded by means of an instrument called the urinometer. It should be allowed to float freely in the fluid in the specimen glass, and the figure is read off from the scale on the instrument, taking the lower level of the meniscus that forms round the stem.

A high specific gravity is found in concentrated urine and also in urine containing sugar.

A dilute urine gives a low specific gravity, a persistently low figure showing inability on the part of the kidneys to concentrate the urine.

Sediment. Normal urine may show a sediment on standing and cooling. This is due to the deposition of urates or phosphates, normal urinary constituents. Urates form a pink or red deposit in urine which is concentrated and acid. If the specimen of urine is gently warmed the sediment will disappear. Phosphates form a white sediment in alkaline or neutral urine. If the urine is acidified by the addition of a few drops of acetic acid the deposit will clear.

Abnormal substances which will form a sediment on standing are pus, mucus and tube casts.

Notes on Urine Testing

Tests for Albumin

Hot Test. Fill two-thirds of a test tube with urine (previously rendered acid if necessary) and boil the top inch over a flame, holding the tube near the bottom. A cloud appears on boiling which may be due to albumin or to phosphates. Add a few drops of dilute acetic acid. If the cloud disappears, it is due to phosphates; if it persists or becomes denser, albumin is present.

Salicyl-sulphonic Acid Test. To 2 inches of urine in a test tube add 10 drops of a 25 per cent. solution of salicyl-sulphonic acid. If albumin is present, the urine in the test tube presents a turbid white appearance.

"Albustix" Reagent Strips. The test end of the strip is dipped in the urine and removed immediately. If no albumin is present the moistened end of the strip shows no colour change, but if protein is present a green or blue-green colour develops at once. Comparison with a colour scale provides a guide to the amount of protein present.

The Use of Esbach's Albuminometer for the Quantitative Estimation of Albumin. The urine must be clear, not too

8*

concentrated and acid in reaction. Therefore, it may be necessary to filter or centrifuge the specimen, to dilute it and to acidify it before making the test. The test tube of the albuminometer is filled to the mark U. with urine and to the mark R. with the reagent (Esbach's reagent is a solution of 10 grammes picric acid and 20 grammes citric acid in 1,000 ml. water). Cork the tube, shake by inverting several times, and set aside for twenty-four hours. The height of the precipitate which forms at the bottom of the tube is read off on the graduated scale and indicates, approximately, grammes of dry albumin per 1,000 parts. Divide the result by 10 to obtain the percentage of albumin and allow for the dilution of the urine if necessary. Esbach's albuminometer should not be allowed to read more than 4 parts per 1,000; if, for example, it shows 10 parts per 1,000 the urine should be diluted. This test is not very accurate and quantitative estimation is usually carried out in the laboratory.

Blood

The presence of blood in the urine is usually visible to the naked eye. The only reliable test for the presence of red blood cells is microscopic examination.

The Guaiacum test for blood pigment is occasionally used.

To 1 inch of urine in a test tube add a few drops of tincture of guaiacum and 1 inch of ozonic ether or ozonic alcohol. If blood is present, a blue ring appears at the junction of the two liquids.

N.B.—A positive reaction is also given by the urine of patients taking iodides.

"Occultest." A sensitive test for the detection of blood in urine is provided by "Occultest" tablets. One drop of well mixed urine from the specimen is placed in the centre of the test paper and one tablet is placed in the centre of the moist area. Two drops of water are then added to the tablet. A positive result is shown by the development of a diffuse area of blue colour appearing on the test paper around the tablet within two minutes.

Sugar

Benedict's Test. Benedict's solution is a solution of sodium carbonate, sodium citrate and copper sulphate. To 1 inch of Benedict's solution in a test tube add not more than 8 drops of urine and boil for two minutes. Allow to cool.

A precipitate which may be greenish-yellow, yellow or orange will appear if sugar be present. Any precipitate appearing after fifteen minutes is of no significance.

"Clinitest" Tablets. "Clinitest" reagent in tablet form is particularly useful for diabetic patients who have to test their own urine at home as the procedure is simple and the results accurate provided that the tablets are fresh. Place 5 drops of urine in a small test tube using a pipette. Rinse the pipette, add 10 drops of water and then drop in one Clinitest tablet. Fifteen seconds after the boiling activity ceases in the test tube shake the tube gently and then compare the colour change with the colour chart provided. The presence of sugar is denoted by a green, greenish brown or orange colour according to the amount present. If an orange colour develops there is 2 per cent. or more of sugar in the specimen.

"Clinistix" Reagent Strips. These strips are impregnated with glucose oxidase and a colour indicator. The test end of a "Clinistix" is dipped in the specimen of urine and removed. If no glucose is present in the specimen of urine no colour change develops in the test strip. If the moistened end turns blue within one minute glucose is present.

Acetone and Diacetic Acid

Rothera's Test. Take an inch of urine in a test tube and saturate it with ammonium sulphate by adding $\frac{1}{2}$ inch of the crystals. Add a small crystal of sodium nitro-prusside or a few drops of a 1 per cent. solution, and then add $\frac{1}{2}$ inch of strong ammonia. The presence of acetone is shown by a violet colour. This colour may not be fully developed for a few minutes.

Crystals of ammonium sulphate and sodium nitro-prusside may be supplied mixed in the right proportions in one bottle.

"Acetest" Tablets. The "Acetest" method is a convenient and accurate test for acetone and diacetic acid. Place 1 tablet on a clean surface, such as a white tile, add 1 drop of urine. Note the colour change at the end of 30 seconds and compare the colour of the tablet with the scale provided. A positive result is shown by a colour change which may vary from a pale lavender to a strong mauve colour.

Bile

Bilirubin

    a. Iodine test. Place some urine in a test tube and add a layer of 10 per cent. iodine solution. A green ring indicates the presence of bile.

    b. "Ictotest" Tablets. Place 5 drops of urine on the test mat provided and one "Ictotest" tablet in the middle of the moist area. Add 2 drops of water to the tablet. A positive result is shown by the development of a bluish-purple area around the tablet.

    c. Fouchet's test. This is a sensitive test for bilirubin which is carried out in the laboratory.

Bile salts

Hay's test. Put some urine in a test tube and sprinkle a little powdered sulphur on the top. The sulphur will sink if bile salts are present owing to the lowered surface tension.

Urobilinogen

Ehrlich's test. To 10 ml. of fresh urine in a test tube add 1 ml. of Ehrlich's solution. Invert the test tube several times to mix the fluids and leave for five minutes. The normal amount of urobilinogen will give a pink colour, abnormal quantities produce a cherry or darker red colour.

Pus

Microscopic examination for pus cells is the best test.

Chlorides

Chlorides, chiefly in the form of sodium chloride, are normal constituents of the urine but the quantity may be diminished in certain diseases and also in excessive loss of salt from the body by other routes.

Fantus Test. Ten drops of urine are measured into the test tube. The pipette is rinsed with distilled water and one drop of potassium chromate solution—the indicator—added. The pipette is rinsed again and then the 2·9 per cent. silver nitrate solution is added a drop at a time and the test tube shaken after the addition of each drop. The end-point is a sharp colour change from yellow to brown. The number of drops needed to produce the end-point gives the concentration of chloride in the urine expressed as grammes of NaCl (sodium chloride) per litre—for example, 5 drops = 5 G. of NaCl per litre. The average normal excretion is 6 G. in 24 hours.

Observation of Stools

In adults the normal stool is solid or semi-solid, brown in colour and formed. The frequency with which a stool is passed varies in different individuals, but the average is once in twenty-four hours.

In infancy the normal stool is yellow and the bowels may act two or three times daily.

Fæces consist of:

> Water.
> Altered bile pigments, which give the normal colour to the stool.
> Bacteria, mostly dead.
> Mucus.
> Cell debris from the intestinal tract.
> Indigestible and undigested food.

Constipation is the condition in which the fæces are passed infrequently and are hard and dry.

Diarrhœa is the condition in which the stools are passed frequently and are fluid.

The bulk of the fæces will to a certain extent depend on the diet; on a mixed diet containing fruit and vegetables there will be a much greater bulk of residue than with a diet containing little residue such as a purely milk diet. Lack of fluids will also reduce the bulk in the large intestine.

In the ordinary healthy individual the bowels are usually opened after the first meal of the day, peristalsis being induced in the large intestine by the activity of the stomach and small intestine after a period of rest.

Note should be taken of the following points with regard to the stool:

(1) Number of times that the bowels are open in twenty-four hours.

(2) Colour, consistency and odour of the stool.

(3) Where an intestinal obstruction or paralytic distension of the intestine is suspected it is also important to note if flatus is passed, as the condition of absolute constipation in which neither fæces nor flatus is passed may be present.

The shape of the stool is probably of little importance, as this is altered by the anal sphincter.

False diarrhœa is the name given to the condition in which the patient has a fluid motion consisting mainly of mucus and very little fæcal matter. This may be noted in cases of carcinoma of the rectum and occasionally in elderly people in whom attention to the bowels has been neglected and a large mass of fæces is impacted in the colon.

Putty-coloured Stools. If for any reason bile cannot enter the intestine, the stool will be light in colour owing to the lack of pigment. The stool will also be fatty owing to the lack of bile, and will have an offensive odour. The patient will probably be constipated.

The presence of undigested fat in the stool is found in jaundice owing to the absence of bile and in diseases of the pancreas where there is a lack of the fat-splitting ferment.

Tarry colour of the stool is due to blood which originates from high up the alimentary tract, either from the stomach or small intestine. The name given to this stool, which is composed almost entirely of digested blood, is "melæna."

Bright blood in the stool indicates bleeding in the lower part of the alimentary tract. The commoner causes are hæmorrhoids or piles, colitis, and carcinoma of the rectum.

Pus in the stool is due to the rupture of an abscess into the rectum or intestine, or to ulcerative colitis.

Mucus may be found in simple irritation of the alimentary tract following some indiscretion in diet or the use of a strong aperient. It may be present in large amounts in colitis and dysentery.

A collection of pus in the abdominal cavity, particularly in the pouch of Douglas, may cause irritation and congestion of the intestinal mucous membrane, and the fact that mucus is noticed in the stool may be the clue to the condition.

Foreign bodies of almost any kind may be swallowed, usually by children and passed in the stool. Such articles may take several days to pass, unless very small, being commonly held up to the pyloric orifice and at the ileo-cæcal junction.

The stools should be sieved until the foreign body has been recovered. The same procedure should be taken following an attack of gall-stone colic, as gall-stones which succeed in passing down the common bile duct into the intestine will be excreted in the stool.

Intestinal Worms. Roundworms, threadworms and tapeworms are the only intestinal parasites at all common in this country. If suspicion of their presence has been aroused, the stool should be collected in a bedpan containing warm water, carefully sieved through black muslin or any suitable thin material and any parasites or segments saved for inspection.

A black colour of the stools is found in patients taking iron or bismuth medicines.

Certain substances are passed along the alimentary tract unchanged, as, for example, barium sulphate used for barium meals and liquid paraffin.

17

Collection of Specimens for Laboratory Investigations

Collection of Material for Laboratory Investigations

EXAMINATION and analysis of body fluids, excreta and tissues may be carried out in order to detect the presence of abnormal substances, an increase or decrease in normal constituents or, following the administration of diagnostic material, to assess the functioning of certain organs.

In a number of conditions bacteriological examination of urine, blood, sputum, serous fluid, and swabs from wounds or from the nose or throat is required in order to identify the infecting micro-organism.

In many cases the collection of specimens and the carrying out of the necessary preliminary preparation of the patient is part of the nurse's responsibility. She should fully understand her part in the investigation and carry out all instructions implicitly and accurately. Should any circumstance arise in which the carrying out of the full instructions becomes impossible, or if any error has been made this should be reported to the ward sister or the medical officer immediately.

The Collection of Specimens

All specimens sent to the laboratory should be as fresh as possible, for in many cases even a few hours' delay will render the specimen unsuitable for examination, due to bacterial decomposition or other causes.

All specimens must be clearly labelled to prevent loss.

Specimens should be collected first thing in the morning before breakfast, the taking of a meal may materially affect the level of some substances in the blood or urine. If it is impossible to collect blood samples before breakfast, an interval of at least 3 hours should be allowed to elapse between the last meal and the collection.

Specimens of Blood

When sending blood for examination the greatest care must be taken to avoid hæmolysis of the specimen, for hæmolysis almost invariably renders it unusable.

To avoid hæmolysis the syringe and needle used must be dry, so sterilizing in a hot air oven is recommended. The container into which the specimen is placed must also be dry and sterile.

For some tests blood serum is required, whilst for others whole unclotted blood must be sent. To prevent clotting potassium oxalate or sodium citrate is added to the specimen. Usually the laboratory supplies tubes with the required quantity of potassium oxalate crystals already added. If, however, these tubes are not available, 1 drop of 20 per cent. potassium oxalate solution should be added to the tube for every 5 ml. or part thereof of blood taken.

The chief exception to this is the blood sugar estimation, where a special tube must be used—this usually contains thymol and fluoride to prevent the disappearance of the sugar, which occurs very rapidly in unpreserved blood. Once the blood has been added to the anticoagulant it must be mixed gently—too vigorous shaking causes hæmolysis—but care must be taken to see that the anticoagulant is thoroughly mixed with the specimen. The specimen container must always be clean, dry and sterile.

Blood Specimens for Clinical Pathology

Bromide ..	..	..	..	10 ml. clotted blood
Calcium ..	..	..	..	*12 ml. clotted blood
Cholesterol	..	..	..	5 ml. oxalated blood
Chloride	..	..	..	7 ml. clotted blood
Carbon dioxide		..	..	*10 ml. heparinized blood
Cold agglutinins..	..	..	..	7 ml. clotted blood
Cross matching	..	..	..	5 ml. clotted blood
Fibrinogen	..	..	..	5 ml. oxalated blood
Flocculation (liver) tests		..	..	7 ml. clotted blood
Gonococcal complement fixation test ..	..	..		7 ml. clotted blood
Kahn tests ..	..	..	..	7 ml. clotted blood

* Special container and syringes for these specimens *must* be obtained from the Laboratory.

Blood Specimens for Clinical Pathology—cont.

Paul-Bunnell tests	..	..	10 ml. clotted blood
Phosphorus	..	..	*7 ml. heparinized blood
Phosphatases	..	..	*5 ml. heparinized blood
Potassium	..	..	*5 ml. heparinized blood
Protein ..	..	..	7 ml. clotted blood
Sodium ..	..	..	*5 ml. heparinized blood
Sugar ..	..	..	1 ml. fluoride blood
Thiocyanate	..	..	7 ml. clotted blood
Urea ..	..	..	5 ml. oxalated blood
Uric acid	..	..	5 ml. oxalated blood
Van den Bergh tests	..	..	7 ml. clotted blood
Wassermann reactions	..	..	7 ml. clotted blood
Widal tests	..	..	7 ml. clotted blood

Blood Counts

Blood counts may be made by drawing blood directly from a finger prick into special pipettes which the operator brings to the bedside. More commonly, however venous blood is collected in an oxalate tube and sent, with two thin blood smears for the differential count to the laboratory for counting. This second method is more convenient, as several other examinations can be made from the same specimen if they are required. Usually 3 ml. are collected.

Normal Values

Red cells per cu. mm.
    Men   4·5–6 million
    Women 4·3–5·5 million

Hæmoglobin, in grammes per 100 ml.
    Men   15–16
    Women   13–15

White cells, per cu. mm.
    5,000–10,000
    Neutrophils   40–60 per cent.
    Lymphocytes 20–40   ,, ,,
    Monocytes   4– 8   ,, ,,
    Eosinophils   1– 3   ,, ,,
    Basophils   0– 1   ,, ,,

* Special container and syringes for these specimens *must* be obtained from the laboratory.

Platelets, per cu. mm.

200,000–500,000

Erythrocyte Sedimentation Rate

The sedimentation rate measures the distance which the red cells fall in one hour when a column of blood is allowed to stand vertically in a glass tube of fine uniform bore. Several different methods are used, and the normal values vary with each method. It is not a diagnostic test, as most infections cause an increase in the rate but it is very useful in following the course of a disease—*e.g.* in rheumatic fever and tuberculosis. The greater the activity of the disease the higher is the sedimentation rate.

Method. Wintrobe's method is the one most commonly used. 3 ml. of blood are placed in a tube containing ammonium and potassium oxalate, and well mixed. A special Wintrobe sedimentation rate tube is then filled and allowed to stand vertically undisturbed for 1 hour, and then the fall in the column of red cells is measured.

Another method is the Westergren method, where 0·4 ml. of a 3 per cent. sodium citrate solution is used for the anti-coagulant and a different size tube is used.

Normal readings

	Men	Women
Wintrobe ..	0 to 9 mm.	0 to 20 mm. in one hour
Westergren ..	3 to 5 mm.	4 to 7 mm. in one hour

Bone Marrow Specimens

Samples of bone marrow may be required in cases of pernicious anæmia and leukæmia. These are obtained by puncturing the manubrium sterni or the iliac crest, see p. 279, and aspirating the bone marrow.

Plasma Proteins

Disturbances of the serum proteins occur in many conditions. Abnormally low levels of serum albumin may give rise to œdema and may be the result of liver diseases, loss of albumin in the urine in the nephrotic syndrome or a diet deficient in proteins.

Serum protein levels are often low in patients with chronic infections or extensive burns.

Bacteriological Examinations

In many conditions specimens are required for bacteriological examination in order to identify the micro-organism responsible.

Materials required for such examinations include:

> throat and nose swabs,
> swabs from wounds,
> sputum,
> urine,
> stools,
> blood,
> pleural and ascitic fluid,
> cerebrospinal fluid.

These specimens must always be collected under strict aseptic conditions and in sterile containers. When taking swabs for bacteriological examination care must be taken to ensure that no antiseptic is applied to the surface for several hours prior to the swabbing. If the patient is under treatment by any chemotherapeutic agent at the time this should be stated.

Specimens will be examined by direct smear and by culture; information can also be obtained with regard to the sensitivity of organisms to the various antibiotics.

Swabs from the Throat and Nose, Wound Swabs

The necessary apparatus ready sterilized is usually obtained from the laboratory and consists of a swab fixed to a short stiff wire or stick, placed inside a test tube and sterilized. For nasopharyngeal examination special swabs in curved glass containers for passing behind the soft palate are supplied.

No antiseptic lotions should be used for swabbing or for gargles for four hours before the swab is taken.

Sputum

The best method is for the patient to expectorate directly into a sterile flask or small container with a screw lid.

If a sputum mug is used, it should be rinsed free from any trace of disinfectant and boiled.

Urine

A catheter specimen of urine (see pp. 257-260) collected in a sterile container is usually required.

Fæces

A freshly passed stool uncontaminated by urine, is required. The specimen is placed in a container which should have a small scoop incorporated in the stopper.

Cerebrospinal Fluid

For complete routine examination 10 to 20 ml. of cerebro-spinal fluid should be sent to the laboratory.

The following points should be borne in mind in collecting these specimens:

contamination with blood detracts from the value of the report in proportion to the amount present;

dilution of the fluid with water, saline, spirits and other fluids must be rigidly avoided;

bacterial contamination invalidates some of the tests such as sugar content and the colloidal gold test.

The fluid is collected by lumbar puncture—see pp. 296–297.

Serous Fluids

Pleural effusions, pericardial effusions and ascitic fluid are formed in a number of conditions.

Microscopic, bacteriological and chemical investigations of these fluids are used to determine the nature of the under-lying disorder.

1. Cell content. In transudates only a small number of cells is present. In pyogenic infections pus cells are present in large numbers, while in tuberculous infection there is a high percentage of lymphocytes. Red blood cells are often present in malignant disease.

2. Bacteriological investigations. In infective conditions culture for pyogenic organisms or the *Mycobacterium tuberculosis* may reveal the organism responsible for the infection. For the detection of tuberculous infection the fluid may be injected into guinea pigs.

3. Chemical examinations. The protein content is increased in infective conditions, but may also be raised to a lesser extent in transudates.

Specimens of Tissues for Histological Examination

Specimens removed at operations should be sent to the laboratory as soon as possible.

Small fragments such as scrapings should not be allowed to become dried.

If the specimen cannot be despatched at once it should be placed for the time in a solution of 10 per cent. formalin in normal saline. Surgical or methylated spirit should not be used.

If sent through the post the nature of the contents should be stated on the label (*i.e.* material for clinical examination) and the parcel marked URGENT. There are special regulations relating to the despatch of specimens through the post, and special containers must be used.

Fractional Test Meal

The activity of the stomach is usually investigated by examining the resting juice and a series of specimens of the contents removed by means of a tube, following stimulation of secretion. In order to standardize conditions, the following procedure is recommended:

Milk and charcoal powder should be taken before retiring.

Next morning, before any food or liquids whatever have been taken a stomach tube is passed and the resting juice is removed as completely as possible and measured. If the position of the patient is changed once or twice complete removal is facilitated.

Stimulation may be effected either by a meal consisting of a gruel made by boiling two table-spoons of oatmeal with a quart of water until the volume is reduced to a pint, or by the injection of histamine.

A sample of 5 to 10 ml. of the contents is then removed through the tube every 15 minutes until no further material is available, usually for 2 to 3 hours.

The patient should be asked not to swallow saliva during the test.

Fermentation must be checked in specimens which have to be sent some distance by the addition to each of a few drops of chloroform or benzene.

Since emotions undoubtedly affect gastric activity, sometimes quite profoundly, steps taken to allay nervousness are well worth while.

The dose of histamine laid down is 0·3 to 0·8 mg. This dose must not be exceeded on account of the great toxicity of histamine. Hypersensitive individuals may show palpitations, generalized flushing, throbbing in head and neck and headache. With the dose laid down, these symptoms are transient and seldom serious. If any alarm is felt, sub-cutaneous injection of 5 to 7 minims of adrenaline will immediately counteract these effects.

The choice of gastric stimulant is decided by the information required. If it is desired primarily to establish the existence or otherwise of complete achlorhydria, the powerful histamine stimulus is better. In most other cases the simple gruel is used. The advantages of both methods may be combined by giving an injection of histamine at the conclusion of the gruel test and removing two or three more samples.

The report consists of a chart giving curves of free hydrochloric and total acidity. The presence or absence of bile, blood, charcoal, lactic acid and starch is also recorded.

The apparatus required consists of:

Ryle's duodenal tube, 10 ml. syringe, and clip for tube.

Lubricant—*e.g.* liquid paraffin.

Specimen bottles—up to 13 are required, size 5 to 10 ml. *One should be marked R.J. (Resting Juice) and the rest numbered from* 1 *onwards.*

Bowl of water.

Two receivers (one for patient).

Mackintosh and dressing towel.

Pint of gruel or injection of histamine should be in readiness.

The patient should be comfortably propped and kept warm.

The bed should be protected with a mackintosh and towel.

Procedure. Lubricate the tube and pass it through mouth or nose. Ask the patient to breathe in and while he is doing so pass the tube a little way. Then ask him to breathe out and swallow. Repeat until the double mark on the tube is level with the teeth, when no more of the tube must be swallowed.

Attach syringe and draw off *all* the resting juice. Get patient to sway about to assist in emptying the stomach completely. Note quantity and report, and also report on any abnormality present. Save all the resting juice if grossly abnormal; otherwise 2 to 5 ml. is sufficient.

(If the tube and resting juice are vomited the latter must be calculated in the total quantity and the tube again passed.)

Give the patient gruel to drink and wait 15 minutes to draw off specimens at 15-minute intervals until stomach is empty. If histamine is ordered instead of gruel the intervals are 30 minutes.

Clear the tube each time by pumping down air until free.

Clip the tube and fasten to the towel round the patient's neck.

Rinse the syringe after collecting each specimen.

To prevent saliva being swallowed give the patient a receiver to spit into, and a towel to wipe mouth.

Remove the tube and give the patient a mouthwash.

Complete absence of free acid is the rule in pernicious anæmia, even after the powerful stimulus of histamine. It has been found that it is impossible to establish the existence of achlorhydria by the examination of a single specimen of gastric juice removed after an hour, since the excretion of free acid often commences later than an hour after the test meal has been taken.

While gastric and duodenal ulcers are often associated with high acid curves, this finding is by no means always indicative of ulcer. A "climbing" curve in which there is no tendency for the acidity to fall is suggestive of pyloric obstruction.

The emptying time of the stomach can be estimated when the gruel test meal is used by the time of disappearance of the starch from the stomach. The presence of charcoal in the resting juice is evidence of greatly delayed emptying time.

Fresh blood is usually due to trauma; blood which has been in the stomach for some time undergoes digestion and imparts a brown colour to the specimen.

Tubeless Test for Free Gastric Acid

A quinine-containing cation exchange resin is given by mouth. If free hydrochloric acid is present in the stomach the quinine is displaced by hydrogen ions, and is absorbed and then excreted in the urine. The following substances must be withheld for 48 hours before the test: all vitamins (except B_{12}), quinine, iron, barium, kaolin and preparations containing aluminium, calcium and magnesium. The patient fasts overnight and breakfast is withheld.

Procedure:

9.00 a.m. The patient empties his bladder, and the urine is discarded. The patient takes the contents of a small Diagnex capsule (caffeine sodium benzoate) well stirred in a glass of water or large cup of tea or coffee without milk or sugar.

9.30 a.m. 0·3–0·8 milligrams of histamine hydrochloride are injected subcutaneously if desired.

10.00 a.m. The patient empties his bladder, and the entire specimen is saved and sent to laboratory labelled "control urine." The patient takes the contents of a large Diagnex capsule (quinine resin granules) well stirred in a glass of water. The granules do not dissolve and should not be chewed; more water may be taken if necessary.

12.00 noon The patient empties his bladder, and the entire specimen is saved and sent to laboratory labelled "test urine."

Interpretation of test. If the 2-hour test urine contains 25 mg. or more of quinine, free hydrochloric acid is present in the stomach; if it contains less than 15 mg. then free acid is absent. If 15–25 mg. of quinine are excreted the test is equivocal and should be repeated; but not before 7 days have elapsed.

NOTE. Renal impairment may interfere with the excretion of the quinine.

Examination of Fæces for Blood

Meat, extracts and soups and very green vegetables—*e.g.* spinach—should be withheld for three days before collecting fæces for this examination; the administration of a purgative on the first of these days is recommended. Patient should not brush his teeth, but should use cotton wool. A sample of ½ to 1 ounce is required.

The report states the result of the benzidene or guaiac test. A positive benzidene test, or guaiac, indicates the presence of blood.

A quick test for the detection of blood in fæces is "Hematest." A thin smear of fæces is placed on the test paper provided, one "Hematest" tablet in the middle of the smear and two drops of water added. A positive result is shown by a diffuse area of blue colour developing around the tablet within two minutes.

Analysis of Fæces for Fat

It is of the greatest importance to inspect specimens of fæces before submitting them for quantitative analysis. The highly fluid stools obtained by means of purgatives and enemas are useless, as also are specimens which are non-homogeneous, unless these are thoroughly mixed to uniform consistency before sending the sample for analysis. It scarcely need be said that oily purgatives and liquid paraffin must not be used for several days before a specimen is sent for fat estimation. On occasions when the whole stool cannot conveniently be forwarded, the material available must be mixed to a uniform consistency and a 1-ounce sample sent in an airtight container.

The report states the percentage of water present, the percentage of the total solids which consists of fat (*i.e.* neutral fat, fatty acid and fatty acid as soap) and the percentage of the total unsplit fat.

Fat Balance Test

The patient is given a standard diet, containing 50 G. fat per day, during the test and for at least 48 hours prior to its commencement. It is important that all the food should be eaten, but if any is left it should be returned to the diet kitchen. Liquid paraffin and oily drugs must not be given during the test, or for at least 3 days prior to its commencement.

Procedure:

7.00 a.m. 1st day. The patient is given 2 capsules of carmine (*i.e.* 1·0 G.) on an empty stomach.

7.00 a.m. 6th day. The patient is given 2 oz. of charcoal in water (*i.e.* 120 hours. later).

Collection of fæces. The stools are examined as passed and those coloured by carmine are saved, as are subsequent stools until the charcoal appears; stools containing charcoal are discarded. The fæces to be saved are transferred completely into a weighed receptacle supplied by the laboratory.

Interpretation of test, normally, 91–99 per cent. of the ingested fat is absorbed.

Pancreatic Function

The internal secretion of the pancreas, insulin, is disturbed in diabetes mellitus, but is not usually affected by other diseases of the pancreas unless the organ has been extensively destroyed. This aspect of pancreatic function is considered under "Carbohydrate Metabolism" on p. 214.

The external secretions of the pancreas may be tested either by estimating the amylase content of the blood or urine or by analyses of the duodenal contents for pancreatic enzymes and bicarbonates.

Urinary Amylase

A 1-ounce sample from a specimen of urine collected over several hours is desirable. When, however it is a matter of urgency, as for example for the confirmation of a diagnosis of acute pancreatitis, examination of a smaller casual specimen is permissible. If the urine has to be sent some distance to the laboratory it should be preserved with benzene.

The normal range of urinary diastase is from 6 to 30 units per ml. A value of 200 or more units in a case with acute abdominal signs is almost certainly due to acute pancreatitis. Intermediate values between 30 and 200, if found regularly may indicate pancreatic duct obstruction.

Duodenal Drainage

A more detailed examination of the pancreatic function may be carried out by examination of the duodenal juice obtained by duodenal drainage. A weighted tube (Rehfuss duodenal tube), see Fig. 44, is passed into the stomach and a specimen of gastric juice is withdrawn. The patient then lies on his right side to promote the passage of the tube into the duodenum. If necessary the position of the tube can be checked by X-ray. When the tube is in the duodenum the contents are aspirated and tested for sodium bicarbonate and the pancreatic enzymes, trypsin, amylase and lipase. Pancreatic secretion may be stimulated by a subcutaneous injection of Mecholyl or an intravenous injection of Secretin.

Liver Function

Tests of liver function are less satisfactory than function tests of some other organs because the liver has numerous functions, any single one of which may be deficient, whilst the others remain relatively intact. Also the liver has a large reserve and has to be very extensively damaged before any of the tests show an abnormal result. No test has yet been devised which tests the liver as a whole, but there are innumerable tests which depend on the different individual functions of the organ. The commonest of these tests are given below.

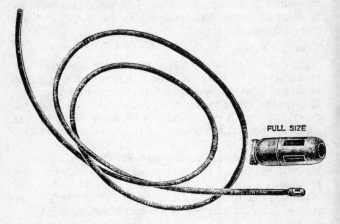

FULL SIZE

FIG. 44.—REHFUSS DUODENAL TUBE.

Bile Pigments

Failure of the liver to excrete bile pigments leads to the accumulation of these in the blood and their excretion in the urine.

Bilirubin. The normal level of bilirubin in the blood serum varies from 0·2 to 0·75 mg. per 100 ml. Increased serum bilirubin is found in liver damage, obstructive jaundice and hæmolytic jaundice.

Bilirubin will be present in the urine in all cases of jaundice except hæmolytic jaundice.

Urobilinogen. This pigment will be present in the urine in cases of incomplete obstructive jaundice, in diffuse liver damage, for example infective hepatitis and in hæmolytic jaundice. In cases of complete obstructive jaundice urobilinogen is absent from the urine.

For urine tests for bile pigments see p. 192.

Serum Protein Tests

These tests are designed to show variations from the normal ability of the liver to synthesize serum proteins. They are not specific tests for liver damage since alterations in the serum proteins may be found in many other diseases.

In liver diseases the serum albumin level is low and the serum globulin is raised. The abnormal composition of the serum proteins is also reflected in the so-called "empirical liver function tests," for example the thymol turbidity and cephalin-cholesterol tests. These become positive when liver function is impaired—*e.g.* in cirrhosis of the liver and infective hepatitis.

Not less than 5 ml. of whole blood is required for each of these tests.

Bromsulphalein Test

This test measures the ability of the liver to excrete a dye, bromsulphalein.

The patient should have a fat-free breakfast and no food thereafter until the test is completed.

Procedure

10.00 a.m. 5 mg. per kilogram of body weight of 5 per cent. bromsulphalein is injected intravenously very slowly over a period of 3 minutes. The ampoule must be warmed if any crystals are visible.

10.45 a.m. 10 ml. of clotted blood is collected from another vein, special care being taken to avoid hæmolysis.

Interpretation of the test. After 45 minutes the serum should show that less than 7 per cent. of the injected dose is still retained.

Prothrombin Concentration Test

Prothrombin is formed in the liver from vitamin K absorbed from the intestine. A low prothrombin may be due to liver damage, or to the non-absorption of vitamin K resulting from biliary obstruction. If the prothrombin concentration is low, the test may be repeated after an injection of vitamin K, and if it then returns to normal it is suggestive of biliary obstruction.

Liver Biopsy

This method of examination is described on p. 298.

Renal Function

Chemical and microscopic examination of the urine, although valuable, gives only limited information as to the condition of the kidneys. Albuminuria, for example, may be met with apart from any nephritic condition, and in nephritis it is not always possible to form an opinion merely from a simple chemical urinary examination, whether the kidneys are functioning properly. Tests have therefore been devised with the object either of directly estimating renal efficiency or of investigating the severity and following the progress of events in a nephritic lesion.

Blood Urea Estimation

Procedure

Breakfast may or may not be taken according to instructions.

8 ml. of blood collected from a vein and treated with potassium oxalate to prevent coagulation is required.

Special tubes containing the correct quantity of potassium oxalate are usually provided on request.

With smaller quantities of blood reasonably satisfactory results can be obtained when the urea content is high, but the results in borderline cases cannot be regarded as sufficiently accurate.

If this test is done in conjunction with a urea concentration test the blood must, of course, be taken before the urea is given.

The normal range of variation of blood urea is from 20 to 40 mg. per 100 ml. Some authorities allow up to 60 mg. in elderly patients. Low values occur in normal pregnancy, but may also be produced by protein deprivation and flushing out the system with water as in diabetes insipidus or diuresis produced by high fluid intake.

Very high results of 100 mg. or more nearly always indicate serious renal impairment, but moderate increases can occur without renal involvement in dehydration, circulatory failure and high protein intake.

Urea Concentration Test (Maclean)

The intake of fluids should be restricted as much as possible from the afternoon preceding the test. No breakfast.

In the morning blood is collected for urea estimation. (See previous test.)

The patient empties the bladder and a sample of this urine is placed in a bottle labelled "1."

15 grammes ($\frac{1}{2}$ ounce) of urea dissolved in about 2 ounces of water is given. A smaller dose is given to children in proportion to age.

At intervals of 1 hour from taking the urea draught the patient empties the bladder.

Three specimens (marked 2, 3 and 4) are obtained in this way. Measure the total quantity of each and send 1 oz. samples to the laboratory. Record the volumes on the labels of the bottles.

It is most important that the blood should be collected *before* the urea draught is given.

Specimens sent from a distance must be preserved by adding a few drops of benzene.

Some authorities prefer to discard the urine passed during the first hour after the draught and consider only the results for the second, third and fourth hours.

Accurate measurements of the time and urine volumes are not necessary.

A figure of 2 per cent. or over in one or more of the hour specimens is regarded as evidence of satisfactory renal function. Diuresis sometimes prevents this concentration being reached and if the volume exceeds 4 ounces (about 120 ml.) a concentration of urea below 2 per cent. does not necessarily indicate poor function. The restriction of fluids is designed to prevent diuresis and ignoring the first hour specimen (in which diuresis is often most marked) also aims at overcoming this difficulty.

Urea Clearance Test

Two methods are used, one without and one with urea, the idea of the latter being to impose a load on the kidneys to provoke maximum efficiency. The need for this is denied by some authorities. In either case the test should be done before breakfast is taken.

First method (without urea):

The patient empties the bladder completely at 8 a.m. Discard this urine.

At 9 a.m. the patient empties the bladder completely.
Place the *whole* specimen directly into a clean bottle
without measurement.   Mark the bottle A.

A specimen of blood is collected immediately for urea
estimation.

At 10 a.m. the patient again empties the bladder completely.
Place the *whole* specimen directly without measurement
into a clean bottle.   Mark the bottle B.

Second method (with urea):

The patient empties the bladder at 8 a.m.   Discard the
urine.   Give immediately a draught containing 15
grammes of urea.   The dose for children varies
according to age.

At 9 a.m. the patient empties the bladder completely.
Discard the urine.

At 9.45 a.m. a specimen of blood is collected for urea
estimation.   (See p. 198.)

At 10 a.m. the patient empties the bladder completely.
Place the *whole* specimen directly without measurement
into a clean bottle.

Greater sensitivity is claimed for this test, but as might be
expected, this increased sensitivity will not be realized in
practice unless close attention is given to detail.

The patient must be asked to make special efforts to empty
the bladder completely at the times specified.

These times must be noted accurately—*i.e.* to the nearest
minute—and recorded on the slip to accompany the specimens for the information of the laboratory.   The intervals
need not be precisely 1 hour if this request is complied with.

All the urine passed must be poured into the specimen
bottles, for the total amount is accurately measured in the
laboratory and any loss of urine will produce a low result.

The specimens of urine must be preserved by the addition
of three or four drops of benzene.

An adequate amount of blood must be sent so that an
accurate determination of the urea can be made.

In the case of children and unusually small or large adults
the height and weight are also required by the laboratory for
the calculation of the result.

Analysis of the specimens submitted gives figures from
which the efficiency of the kidneys is calculated, the result

being in terms of the percentage of average normal renal function. The common range in normal health is from 75 to 120 per cent.

Urine Concentration Test

No fluids are allowed from 4 p.m. on the preceding day until 8 a.m. on the morning of the test. The patient empties his bladder at 8, 9 and 10 a.m. and the volume and specific gravity of each specimen is measured. The specific gravity of at least one specimen should exceed 1,025 if renal function is normal. This test should not be done if the blood urea is raised.

Water Elimination Test

The patient should remain in bed during the test. No food or fluid is allowed after 8 a.m. The bladder is emptied at 8 a.m. and the patient then drinks 1,200 ml. of water within half an hour. The bladder is emptied at 9, 10 and 11 a.m. and at 12 noon. The volume and specific gravity of each specimen is measured.

If the renal function is normal at least 1,000 ml. of urine is excreted within the four hour period and the specific gravity of at least one specimen should fall to 1,003 or less.

The ability of the kidneys to excrete the full amount of urine is impaired not only in renal disease but also in Addison's disease, in this disease the excretion of urine will be found to have returned to normal after the administration of cortisone.

Phenolsulphonphthalein Test

An intravenous injection of a dye, phenolsulphonphthalein 1 ml., is given. On the day before a catheter is passed and left *in situ*. For the test the following are required:

1 ml. syringe.
Wide-necked glass bottles 2 or 3, size approximately 10 ounces, with good stoppers or corks.
One table-spoon of bicarbonate of soda is put in each bottle.

The intravenous injection is given and the urine is allowed to drain by catheter into the first bottle for 1 hour. The time at which the pink coloration appears must be carefully checked and written down—normally it is in 3 to 4 minutes.

First bottle drains for 1 hour and is marked "First Hour."
Second bottle drains for 1 hour and is marked "Second Hour."

The third bottle is for use only if the patient secretes more urine within 1 hour than one bottle can hold.

Care must be taken to collect a full hour's specimen, and the bottle or bottles must be marked accordingly.

From these specimens the amount of dye excreted in each of the hours is estimated. Over the total 2-hour period 60 per cent. or more of the dye injected should be excreted.

Renal Biopsy, see p. 299. see p. 299.

Carbohydrate Metabolism

The following tests are used to detect disturbances of carbohydrate metabolism, in particular in diabetes.

Estimation of Blood Sugar

This is usually carried out in the early morning before food has been taken.

If the patient is unable to visit the laboratory, $\frac{1}{2}$ ml. of blood may be sent in a small tube (supplied on request) containing a special preservative mixture. The tube must be shaken thoroughly to mix the blood with the preservative. Blood without this preservative powder (5 parts sodium fluoride, 1 part powdered thymol) is useless for this test, as the sugar content begins to diminish within an hour. Blood from a vein may be sent from cases which do not bleed freely after puncture of a finger or the lobe of the ear. The great majority of normal fasting blood-sugar values lie between 80 to 120 mg. per 100 ml.

Glucose Tolerance Test

The way in which an individual is able to deal with a standard quantity of sugar affords valuable information as to the presence, or otherwise, of a diabetic tendency. It is desirable that the test should be done in the morning before food has been taken. Extremes of high or low carbohydrate diet should be avoided for at least one day before the test. Nervous tension and rush before and during the test should be discouraged and smoking must be forbidden.

The patient may be sent to the laboratory by appointment

for the test or, where this is not practicable the following procedure is adopted:

> The patient empties the bladder. A sample of this urine is placed in a bottle marked A.
>
> A 0·5 ml. sample of blood is collected in a special blood-sugar tube.
>
> 50 grammes of glucose dissolved in 100 ml. of water (about 4 ounces) is given, by mouth. For children a smaller dose according to age is given.
>
> At ½-hour intervals thereafter, five more samples of blood are collected.
>
> The patient empties the bladder one hour and two hours after the administration of glucose. Place these specimens in bottles labelled "B" and "C."

When the urine specimens are sent from a distance to the laboratory for testing they should be boiled or preserved with a few drops of benzene to ensure sterility. Chloroform must *not* be used since it gives rise to reducing substances.

Normally the test should show a fasting sugar between 80 and 120 mg. per 100 ml., a definite rise during the first hour and a return to fasting limits within 2 hours. The maximum reading should not exceed 180 mg. per 100 ml. and no sugar should be found in the specimens of urine.

Calcium Metabolism

The commoner causes of disturbed calcium metabolism are diseases of the parathyroid glands and failure of absorption of calcium due to steatorrhœa or vitamin D deficiency and chronic renal disease.

In the condition of hyperparathyroidism due to tumours of the parathyroid glands calcium is lost from the bones leading to osteomalacia and a raised serum calcium level. In these cases the blood phosphorus is low and the alkaline phosphatase level in the blood is raised. In tetany due to absence of the parathyroid hormone blood calcium is low.

In steatorrhœa there is failure of absorption of calcium from the gut which gives rise to low blood calcium and osteomalacia.

The administration of vitamin D aids calcium absorption, but excessive dosage can cause a raised level of the blood calcium.

Laboratory tests used in disordered calcium metabolism include the following:

1. Estimation of the blood calcium.
2. Estimation of the blood phosphorus.
3. Estimation of the blood alkaline phosphatase.
4. Calcium balance estimation.

This latter test involves a somewhat complicated routine as detailed in the following instructions.

Calcium Balance Routine

The patient is on a weighed and analysed diet. The tray is delivered to the patient and collected by the dietician, who weighs any rejects. The diet is the same throughout the test. The whole of it must be eaten. Nothing extra is allowed.

The water is distilled for drinking. As much as the patient likes may be given. All food is cooked in distilled water in utensils kept solely for this purpose. No toothpaste may be used, distilled water mouthwashes are substituted.

The patient is on this routine for 6 days before collections are begun. This is the equilibrium period during which time small alterations may be made in the diet to suit the patient's taste.

At 6 a.m. on the first day of the specimen collection, the patient empties the bladder. This urine is rejected. All subsequent specimens are collected in 24-hourly bottles, the last specimen of each 24 hours being obtained at 6 a.m. after which a new bottle is begun. Each bottle contains 10 ml. toluol to preserve the urine.

The evening before the start of the collections a carmine cachet is given to colour the faeces. This is given the evening before the end of each balance period. Following this all stools are saved in individual containers and the balance periods are considered to be from the end of the marked (red) stool to the end of the second marked stool.

Urine and faeces must be collected separately. The bed-pan is rinsed in distilled water before being used by patient. After use it is cleaned in the normal way and rinsed in distilled water again. All the faeces passed must be saved. The bedpan is lined with cellophane to facilitate this.

No drugs may be given unless charted. All drugs given

must be analysed. The advisability of giving any drug should be checked before administration.

This routine may be modified to allow balance tests on other substances to be carried out.

Phosphatase

Two forms of phosphatase enzyme are present in blood serum, the alkaline and the acid. The former is increased in bone diseases, such as hyperparathyroidism bone tumours and Paget's disease; the latter is frequently increased in carcinoma of the prostate gland with secondary deposits. The laboratory should be told which form is required when sending the specimen.

Either form of phosphatase can be determined on the serum obtained from 5 to 6 ml. of blood. The normal ranges vary with the method used for determination, and information will be given by the laboratory.

Tests of Thyroid Gland Function

Basal Metabolic Rate

At complete physical and mental rest a healthy individual consumes a definite volume of oxygen per minute, the actual amount depending mainly on the sex, age, height and weight.

During the test the patient lies quietly on a bed and breathes through wide rubber tubes into a special apparatus which records the respirations over a measured period of time, usually 6 minutes.

From the recording so made the volume of oxygen used by the patient can be measured. This is compared with the volume used by a normal subject of the same sex, age height and weight.

Endocrine disorders, more especially those involving the thyroid and pituitary, profoundly alter this basal metabolism, and hence its determination is not infrequently of considerable value in detecting the existence and assessing the severity of conditions of this nature.

The B.M.R. is considered normal if the figure obtained is within -10 to $+15$ per cent. of the value predicted for the individual in question. Success depends almost entirely on the patient being perfectly quiet and at ease; he must go without breakfast and should relax completely for about half an hour before the test is begun. This must be achieved without fuss about the test itself. In order to allay apprehension the simple nature of the procedure and its object should be explained, or, better still, demonstrated beforehand.

Radioactive Iodine

A tracer dose of radioactive iodine (I_{131}) is given orally or occasionally intravenously, and the amount of "take up" or concentration of the radioactive material by the thyroid gland is recorded by a Geiger counter sited over the thyroid area.

The results of the test may be invalidated if the patient is given radiological contrast media or food containing iodine, thyroid preparations, perchlorates or thiocyanates, or radioactive isotopes. Some of these preparations may affect the result of the test even if a considerable time elapses between their discontinuation and the test, as for example Lugol's iodine and contrast media; it is therefore advisable to have an interval of 4 weeks if at all possible before carrying out the test.

The following instructions should be given to the patient:

1. No fish should be eaten for at least 2 days before coming for this test.
2. Iodized throat tablets, cough linctus and any proprietary food said to have a high iodine content should also be avoided. If these have been taken during the past month, will you please inform the department at the time of making the appointment.
3. A light breakfast may be taken on the morning of test.

18

Oxygen Therapy

OXYGEN benefits the patient whose respiratory capacity is diminished, as is the case following chest injuries or operations on the lung, in pneumonia, acute pulmonary œdema, cardiac failure and many other conditions.

Oxygen Cylinders and Fittings

For purposes of identification oxygen and other medical gas cylinders are painted in distinctive colours and the name and/or symbol of the gas is stencilled on the cylinder. Oxygen cylinders are painted black with a white valve end.

Oxygen is compressed into cylinders of different sizes at 132 atmospheres, which is an equivalent of approximately 1,940 lb. per square inch. This pressure must be reduced prior to administration to a patient. Wherever possible an automatic oxygen regulator should be employed for this purpose, but when not available a fine adjustment valve may be used with care. A litre gauge or flowmeter is necessary in order that the prescribed rate of flow may be maintained. These gauges may be of the dial or the bobbin type. In the latter a bobbin inside a graduated glass tube rises as the oxygen passes through and the height of the bobbin against the scale shows the amount of oxygen being delivered. The flowmeter is usually incorporated in the cylinder fitting with the pressure gauge and regulator.

Before attaching the regulator to the cylinder the cylinder valve should be opened slightly, so that any grit or dust that may have accumulated may be blown out. The regulator is then fitted into the head of the cylinder by inserting the threaded end into the valve opening and tightening it by means of the winged nut. The litre gauge should be turned off and the cylinder opened slowly until the cylinder contents gauge shows "full," the cylinder is then opened completely by giving the key one more turn. The cylinder is then ready for use.

In some wards the oxygen supply may be delivered by a pipe-line to each bed, but every ward should possess at least one oxygen outfit ready for immediate use. The cylinder, in a wheeled stand with the fittings and the apparatus for

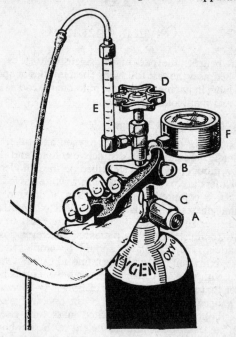

FIG. 45.—AN OXYGEN CYLINDER FITTED WITH A FINE ADJUSTMENT VALVE.

The illustration shows: A, Main tap for turning on flow of oxygen; B, Wing nut for attaching regulator, etc., to the cylinder (this nut may be loosened with a special spanner); C, Lock nut; D, Fine adjustment valve; E, Flowmeter; F, Pressure guage.

delivering the oxygen to the patient, should be regarded as emergency apparatus which must always be kept in working order. An empty cylinder should be clearly marked "EMPTY" when removed from the stand and should be replaced at once by a full cylinder.

Fire Precautions

Although oxygen itself does not burn, any material which burns in atmospheric air will burn much more easily if the concentration of oxygen in the air is increased. Therefore certain precautions should be strictly observed.

Patients and visitors should be warned against smoking or lighting matches in the vicinity. No electrical bells, lights or heating pads should be allowed inside an oxygen tent and children should not be given mechanical toys. The patient must not be rubbed with oil or spirit whilst the tent is being operated; should such procedure be necessary the oxygen flow must be discontinued during the time that the treatment is being carried out.

Oil or grease of any description must not be used on the oxygen cylinder or fittings. The nozzle of the cylinder must be cleaned before attaching the regulator.

The "B.L.B." (Boothby, Lovelace and Bulbulian) Apparatus (Fig. 46). This apparatus consists of a rubber mask joined by a metal connecting device to a thin rubber bag similar to a football bladder. The usual type of mask is the oronasal one. The mask is fastened round the head by a rubber strap. Two tubes leading from the sides of the nose-piece pass round the sides of the mouth, joining over the chin to form a single tube to which the metal tube connecting with the breathing bag is attached. The connecting tube is fitted with an inlet tube for the oxygen. With a flow of oxygen at the rate of 7 litres per minute an alveolar concentration of 90 per cent. oxygen can be attained. The rubber bag has a capacity of about 700 ml., and should always be slightly distended while the apparatus is in use. When the patient breathes out, the expired air enters the bag and is mixed with the incoming oxygen. When the patient inspires, the mixture of air and oxygen in the bag passes through the connecting tube into the mask.

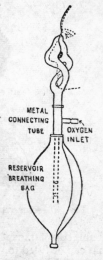

METAL CONNECTING TUBE

OXYGEN INLET

RESERVOIR BREATHING BAG

FIG. 46.—"B.L.B." APPARATUS.

9*

The face piece should be tried on the patient and the necessary adjustments made to the position and length of the straps before the mask is attached to the tubing connecting with the cylinder.   Unless the situation is urgent a little time should be spent in familiarizing the patient with the appearance and the feel of the mask.

The B.L.B. apparatus has great advantages over the older types of oxygen masks, patients quickly become accustomed to wearing it and tolerate it well, also nursing procedures can be carried out without interrupting the treatment.   The nasal type of mask allows the patient to eat and drink and also to expectorate.   If, however, the patient cannot breathe through his nose or cannot co-operate in the treatment the oronasal type of mask must be used.

Polythene Mask

This type of mask is very light in weight and also has the advantage of being inexpensive and can be destroyed after use, thus presenting no problem of sterilization.   It consists of a

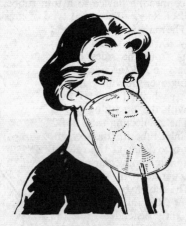

FIG. 47.—DISPOSABLE POLYTHENE MASK (POLYMASK).

double bag of transparent polythene with a flexible wire frame that can be fitted to the patient's face.   It is kept in position by thin cords on each side which hitch the bag to the patient's ears.   Oxygen passes from the cylinder between the layers of the bag and reaches the patient through two small holes in the inner layer, there are also ventilation holes in the outer layer. Some patients however find the polythene mask, in spite of its lightness, less comfortable than a well-fitting B.L.B. mask.

Oxygen Tent

There are several types of oxygen tents in use, but the general principles of construction and the management of the patient in the tent are very similar.

The aim is to have an oxygen content of 40 to 60 per cent. (average concentration 50 per cent.) inside the tent. The excess carbon dioxide must be removed, and the air prevented from becoming over-hot and excessively humid. The tent

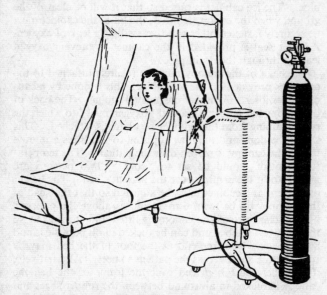

FIG. 48.—OXYGEN TENT (OXYGENAIRE).

is made of transparent plastic material attached to a frame; the whole is mounted on wheels, enabling the tent to be easily moved. The windows in the front of the tent are made of transparent celluloid. The front flap is fitted with two sleeve openings, through which the nurse's arms can be put to feed or give other attention to the patient. Cooling of the air inside the tent is effected by passing the air through an ice box, and in some types of tents the carbon dioxide is removed by passing the air through a container of soda-lime.

A full cylinder of oxygen ready for use, as described above, and a supply of ice should be obtained before erecting the tent. A wall thermometer will also be required. This is hung in the tent when it is erected, at the opposite end to the ice cabinet.

The ice is broken into pieces about the size of a man's fist and the ice container filled to capacity. About 3 feet of rubber tubing is then connected to the water outlet of the ice cabinet and a pail is placed under the rubber drain pipe. The ice cabinet is raised so that it will be clear of the ground when the canopy is fitted; the lid of the cabinet must be securely fastened otherwise there will be a leak of oxygen. A water seal is provided in the cabinet to prevent oxygen leaking through the drain pipe.

The head of the canopy must be securely attached to the openings provided on the ice cabinet, this is done by means of rubber inserts or rubber corrugated tubing. The back of the canopy has a nozzle marked "oxygen inlet" to which the rubber tubing from the cylinder regulator is attached. This should be done and the flow adjusted to five litres a minute before the canopy is placed over the patient. The temperature control should be set to "cold." Two persons are needed to fit the canopy over the patient's bed. The height of the tent and cabinet must be adjusted so that the head of the canopy will be from 6 to $1\frac{1}{2}$ inches above the patient's head. The skirt of the canopy is lifted and spread out so that it covers the bed and can be tucked in on both sides and at the back. The free end at the foot of the bed may be rolled into a sheet across the patient's knees. Alternatively, if a rubber sheet is placed over the frame of the bed the canopy is tucked in all round between the rubber sheet and the mattress. The sleeve openings of the canopy are sealed by rolling them up and securing the flaps with bulldog clips.

Once the tent is set up the oxygen flow should be turned on until the needle of the litre gauge registers "flush" and this full flow is then allowed to continue for about 5 minutes, after which time the flow is reduced to the dosage ordered, which may be from 4 to 8 litres per minute.

Whenever the sleeves have to be opened to allow access to the patient the tent should be flushed with oxygen for five minutes after the apertures have been closed. This is also necessary if the canopy has to be untucked. The temperature should be maintained at 65° to 70° F. and to do this the ice cabinet must be kept full by adding ice at frequent intervals. In warm weather it may be necessary to add ice at least every hour.

Some tents have an electric motor incorporated which forces the oxygen to circulate and allows greater control of the temperature and improves the ventilation inside the tent.

Although oxygen tents are very suitable for the treatment of infants and young children for whom face masks are not practical, recent investigation into the cause of blindness occurring in premature infants has shown that high concentrations of oxygen can cause blindness. Caution is therefore necessary in the administration of oxygen to these infants and it is recommended that a concentration of 40 per cent. should not be exceeded.

Nasal Tubes

This method is used if a tent is not available or a face mask is not suitable, as, for example, where there are facial injuries. It is much less efficient than either the tent or the mask as it is wasteful of oxygen and the patient cannot as a rule tolerate a rate of flow greater than 4 litres per minutes. Three types of apparatus can be used:

1. A bifurcated metal tube with two pieces of soft rubber tubing attached. The metal tube is carried by a head piece and webbing band which is fastened round the patient's head.

2. A spectacle frame which carries two pieces of rubber tubing and is worn by the patient in the same way as an ordinary pair of spectacles.

3. Two soft rubber catheters connected by a Y-shaped connection to the delivery tube from the oxygen apparatus.

When giving oxygen by nasal tubes it is necessary to moisten the oxygen by passing it through a humidifier before it reaches the patient, as dry oxygen is irritating to the nasal passages.

Before the tubes are inserted the nostrils should be cleaned with warm boracic lotion and wool swabs.   A cocaine spray or cocaine ointment may be used in order to make the treatment less uncomfortable for the patient.   The two nasal tubes should be passed about 2 inches along the floor of the nostrils.   The tubes should be removed and cleaned if left in for more than twenty-four hours.

19

Fluid and Electrolyte Balance

THE total quantity of water in the body amounts to approximately 60 per cent. of the body weight. Two thirds of this is inside the cells, the so-called intracellular fluid, while the remaining one third is extracellular. Of the extracellular fluid about a quarter is contained inside the blood vessels as circulating blood plasma. The remaining three quarters make up the interstitial fluid. An adult weighing 70 kg. thus contains a total of about 42 litres of water of which 28 litres are intracellular and 14 extracellular. The latter consists of about 3·5 litres of plasma and 10·5 litres of interstitial fluid.

The electrolytes* present in these fluid compartments can be divided into the basic cations sodium (Na), potassium (K), calcium (Ca) and magnesium (Mg), and the acid anions chloride (Cl), bicarbonate (HCO₃), phosphate (PO₄) and sulphate (SO₄). Potassium and phosphate are present in large quantities in the intracellular fluid while sodium and chloride predominate in the extracellular fluid.

The composition of the extracellular fluid can be determined by the estimation of its various components in the blood plasma and disturbances of electrolyte balance can thus be assessed. In health the total quantity of water in each compartment and its electrolyte composition remains remarkably constant.

Daily Requirements

An adult loses about 1 litre of water daily through the lungs, skin and fæces and should excrete at least 1 litre in the

---

*Electrolytes are substances which in solution become electrically charged; these charged particles are known as "ions" and can bring about chemical changes. Electrolytes which carry a positive charge are called cations, those which carry a negative charge are known as anions.

urine so that the minimum daily requirement of water is 2 litres. In addition he requires about 3·5 G. (60 m.Eq.) of sodium chloride. These quantities can be given intravenously as 2 litres of 5 per cent. glucose in 1/5th normal saline. The glucose serves as a source of calories. For short periods health can be maintained without administration of potassium but if food has to be withheld for more than a few days 2 G. (50 m.Eq.) of potassium should be given daily preferably by mouth in the form of 4 G. of potassium chloride or 30 ml. (1 oz.) of Mixture of Potassium Citrate, N.F. If the patient is febrile and is sweating profusely the fluid intake will have to be increased. Additional quantities of water and electrolytes will have to be given if these are being lost through vomiting, diarrhœa, gastro-intestinal aspirations or polyuria. Allowances must also be made for any losses which may have occurred before treatment is started. Careful intake and output charts and repeated electrolyte estimations are needed to control intravenous therapy.

Disturbances of Fluid and Electrolyte Balance

In practice these disturbances are usually multiple, affecting the water content and several of the electrolytes simultaneously.

1. Water

a. Water depletion or dehydration is the result of either excessive loss due to vomiting, diarrhœa or polyuria or of insufficient intake often due to coma. It is characterized clinically by severe thirst and a dry tongue. It can be corrected by intravenous administration of 5 per cent. glucose in water.

b. Excess of water or water intoxication is usually due to the administration of excessive amounts of fluids to patients suffering from anuria. It leads to œdema, lethargy, mental confusion and ultimately convulsions. It can be avoided by restricting the daily fluid intake of patients with anuria or oliguria to 1 litre of water plus the volume of urine passed during the previous 24 hours. If severe, it can be treated by making the patient sweat and by the intravenous administration of hypertonic (5 per cent.) saline.

2. Sodium

a. Sodium depletion may occur as the result of prolonged vomiting, gastric or intestinal aspirations, diarrhœa, excessive sweating or excessive urinary loss of salt as in diabetic ketosis, Addison's disease and some cases, of chronic nephritis. It is characterized by inelasticity of the skin, low intra-ocular pressure and, in severe cases, a low blood pressure and shock. It can be corrected by the oral administration of salt or by normal saline intravenously. In more severe states of depletion, hypertonic (2 per cent. or 3 per cent.) saline may be used.

b. Common causes of sodium excess are cardiac failure, some forms of renal disease such as the nephrotic syndrome and the excessive administration of cortisone. It is characterized by œdema and can be treated by restricting the salt intake and by giving mercurial diuretics or ion exchange resins.

3. Potassium

a. Potassium deficiency (hypokalæmia) may be due to a low intake, persistent vomiting, chronic diarrhœa, chronic renal disease polyuria due to diabetic ketosis, excessive administration of cortisone and rarely due to adrenal tumours secreting aldosterone. It causes muscular weakness and paralysis and changes in the electrocardiogram. It can be treated by giving potassium, preferably by mouth, as potassium chloride or citrate. 15 ml. ($\frac{1}{2}$ oz.) of Mixture of Potassium Citrate, N.F., contains 3 G. of potassium citrate or 28 m.Eq. of potassium. Potassium can be given intravenously as a 0·2 per cent. or 0·3 per cent. solution of potassium chloride but this should be done only if there is an adequate urinary output and the rate of administration should not exceed 1 litre in 4 hours owing to the danger of hyperkalæmia.

b. Potassium excess (hyperkalæmia) occurs in anuria, renal failure and in Addison's disease. It may cause cardiac arrest. To prevent hyperkalæmia it is essential in cases of anuria or renal failure to avoid the administration of any potassium.

4. Bicarbonate (HCO_3)

Changes in the HCO_3 content of the plasma reflect disturbances of the acid-base balance.

a. Acidosis. In this condition there is a tendency for the blood to become more acid than normal due to an excess of acid anions over basic cations. This may occur as the result of the formation of acids such as ketones in diabetic ketosis, the administration of acid forming substances such as salicylates or failure of excretion of acid metabolites in renal failure. It is also caused by the loss of sodium and potassium through diarrhœa or intestinal aspirations.

In these conditions the plasma HCO_3 will be low and, unless there is renal failure, the urine will be acid. Acidosis causes hyperventilation and, if severe, it leads to mental confusion and coma.

Treatment consists of appropriate therapy of the underlying condition, *e.g.* the administration of insulin in diabetic ketosis, and the administration of sodium bicarbonate or sodium citrate by mouth if the patient is not vomiting, or intravenously as normal saline. The chloride ions will be excreted by the kidneys if renal function is normal and the sodium ions will be retained. Alternative solutions for intravenous use are ⅙th molar sodium lactate or saline lactate with or without potassium.

Acidosis can also be due to retention of carbon dioxide in chronic lung disease such as emphysema, so-called respiratory acidosis. In this condition the plasma bicarbonate is raised but the reaction of the urine is acid.

b. Alkalosis. Here there is a tendency for the blood to become more alkaline than normal due to an excess of basic cations over acid anions. It is due either to excessive and prolonged administration of alkalies or to the loss of hydrochloric acid through persistent vomiting as in pyloric stenosis or gastric aspiration.

The plasma bicarbonate will be raised and the urine will be alkaline unless there is renal failure which may develop as the result of long-standing alkalosis. Clinically it is characterized by anorexia, mental confusion and sometimes tetany.

It can be corrected by intravenous administration of normal saline, chloride being retained by the kidneys in excess of sodium. Long-standing cases of alkalosis are often complicated by potassium depletion which will have to be corrected simultaneously.

Respiratory alkalosis may occur as the result of loss of CO_2 due to overbreathing. It is characterized by a low plasma HCO_3 in association with an alkaline urine and may give rise to tetany.

20

Intravenous and Subcutaneous Infusions: Transfusion of Blood and Plasma

Intravenous Infusion

THE indications for the use of intravenous infusion of saline or glucose-saline and other electrolytic solutions in the restoration and maintenance of fluid and electrolyte balance have been described in the preceding chapter.

Isotonic electrolyte solutions, *e.g.* Darrow's sodium potassium chloride lactate solution or dilute plasma with potassium chloride, are given intravenously in the treatment of dehydration in infants. Electrolyte solutions may also be given in the treatment of uræmia and diabetic coma. In these cases the solutions are individually prescribed and carefully checked by blood examination. Hypertonic salt solutions, 10 or 15 per cent. sodium chloride, are occasionally used with the object of relieving intracranial tension in cerebral cases.

The same apparatus as that used for the transfusion of blood or plasma is suitable. The instruments for cutting down on a vein and tying in a cannula should be provided.

In all intravenous infusions a careful record of the fluid given by this and other routes and of the fluid output from the patient must be kept.

Blood and Plasma Transfusion

The usual indications for transfusion of blood or plasma are severe hæmorrhage, burns and shock. Transfusion with whole blood or "packed red cells" is also often required in the treatment of chronic anæmia, as for example from repeated small blood losses.

The standard transfusion fluids provided by the Blood Transfusion Services of the United Kingdom are:

1. Whole blood.

2. Dried plasma or serum, with sterile pyrogen-free fluid for reconstitution.
3. Concentrated suspension of red cells ("packed red cells").

There are also a number of plasma substitutes which are widely used—*e.g.* dextran, a polysaccharide, and gelatin solutions.

Blood Groups

Transfusion of blood from one person to another is fraught with great risks unless it can be proved that the blood of the donor is compatible with the blood of the recipient.   Human blood can be classified into one of four main categories dependent on the presence in the red cells of substances known as A and B agglutinogens.

The four groups of human blood are:

Group A.   This group has A agglutinogens in the red cells and anti-B agglutinin in the blood plasma.

Group B.   This group has B agglutinogens in the red cells and anti-A agglutinin in the plasma.

Group AB.   This group has both A and B agglutinogens in the cells but no anti-agglutinins in the plasma.

Group O.   This group has no agglutinogens in the cells but both anti-A and anti-B agglutinins in the plasma.

Group A therefore cannot receive blood from Group B as the B group has anti-A agglutinins.

Group B similarly cannot receive from Group A since B group blood contains anti-A agglutinins.

Group AB has no anti-agglutinins and can therefore receive blood from all other groups ("universal recipient" group).

Group O has both anti-A and anti-B agglutinins, therefore can only receive blood from O group, but has no A and B agglutinogens and can therefore be given to all other groups ("universal donor" group) as the red cells of the donor's blood will not be agglutinated by the recipient's plasma.

It is now known that there are sub-types of the various groups and typing blood in its main group is not sufficient to ensure compatibility between the donor's blood and that of recipient.   For this reason direct cross-matching of a sample of blood from the patient with the blood to be used for the transfusion is carried out as a routine procedure, even though the groups to which the two belong is known.

In 1940 the presence of another agglutinogen in human blood, the rhesus or Rh factor was discovered; the name denotes the fact that this substance is found also in the blood cells of the rhesus monkey. Eighty-five per cent. of the population have this factor and are therefore classed as Rh positive; the remaining 15 per cent. are Rh negative and may form an agglutinin against the Rh factor if Rh positive blood is introduced into their blood stream.

The Rh factor is of importance when blood transfusions are undertaken under certain conditions. If Rh positive blood is given to a Rh negative patient anti-Rh agglutinins may be formed by the recipient's blood and if a further transfusion is given, even some years later, a transfusion reaction can be caused. The Rh factor is also of importance in pregnancy. A woman with Rh negative blood may have a Rh positive infant and this may result in the formation of anti-Rh agglutinins in the mother's plasma. The filtration of the agglutinins from the mother's blood can destroy the fœtal red cells and lead to the condition known as "erythro-blastosis fœtalis" with severe anæmia and jaundice. The condition is also dangerous to the mother should she require a blood transfusion; if Rh positive blood is used a severe reaction will occur.

The bottles of blood supplied by the Blood Transfusion Service are labelled with the ABO and Rh groups, date of collection and date after which it is unfit for use.

Whole blood may be used up to 21 days after withdrawal. Red cells suspensions must be used within 24 hours after the preparation of the suspension.

Test for Blood Group. In order to determine to which of the four groups, AB, A, B or O, an individual may belong, stock sera of groups A and B are used. In addition, direct matching of the serum of the recipient against the red cells of the potential donor is carried out whenever possible.

Requirements for blood grouping test:

Stock sera of Groups A and B.
Microscope slide or a white tile.
Cetrimide, ether or spirit.
Swabs.

A large bayonet-pointed suture needle (sterile).

A sterile 2-ml. syringe and hypodermic needle for venipuncture.

Small test tubes.

Normal saline or sodium citrate solution for diluting the blood.

For grouping with the stock sera only two or three drops of blood are needed and can be obtained by pricking the skin. For the direct matching test about 1 ml. of blood is required and this is withdrawn from a vein.

Requirements for Taking Blood from a Donor

The standard "taking set" consists of:

A pint-sized sterile vacuum bottle containing 120 ml. of anticoagulant solution, consisting of 1·66 per cent. disodium hydrogen citrate and 2·5 per cent. glucose.

Two pieces of tubing: one is packed with cotton wool and has a stainless steel needle at one end which is pushed through the rubber diaphragm closing the bottle and acts as an air vent; the second and longer tubing has a needle at both ends, one needle is pushed through the rubber diaphragm and the other is the taking needle for insertion into the donor's vein.

A sphygmomanometer or piece of rubber tubing to act as a tourniquet.

2 ml. syringe, needles and local anæsthetic.

Gallipot containing surgical spirit, cetrimide or other suitable skin cleanser.

A packet containing sterile swabs, towels and small dressings.

Adhesive strapping.

A mackintosh.

A bowl of cold water or cold sodium citrate solution for the needle and tubing after use.

Receptacle for used swabs.

A roller bandage for the donor to grasp.

The donor should lie on a couch of convenient height with his arm bared to the shoulder and the elbow extended. The sphygmomanometer cuff is applied well above the elbow and pumped up to a pressure of 80 mm. The skin is cleaned and the local anæsthetic injected.

The donor is given the roller bandage to hold. When the needle has entered the vein the doctor will require the nurse to rotate the bottle gently in order to mix the blood with the sodium citrate solution in the bottle. The patient may be asked to clasp and unclasp his hand over the bandage to

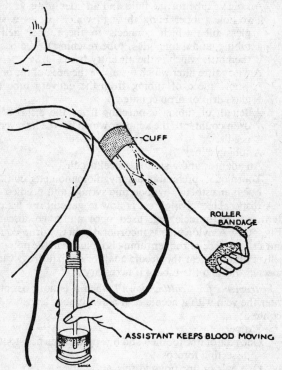

CUFF

ROLLER BANDAGE

ASSISTANT KEEPS BLOOD MOVING

FIG. 49.—COLLECTING BLOOD FROM DONOR.

increase the flow of blood from the vein. When the blood has been withdrawn the sphygmomanometer cuff is removed and the needle withdrawn. A few ml. of blood from the tubing are run into a small bottle to be used for testing and checking the blood group. Firm pressure is made over the puncture and a small dressing applied. The donor should remain lying on the couch for ten minutes and then be given a large cup of sweetened tea or coffee. After a further rest of quarter-of-an-hour he may be allowed to leave.

Requirements for Giving Blood

The bottle containing the citrated blood, with a metal band and handle for suspension to the transfusion stand.

An outlet tube for the fluid and an inlet or air-vent.

Two-hole rubber bung through which passes a short glass tube which connects to the rubber delivery tubing, and a long glass tube reaching to the base of the bottle which is the air entry tube.

A wire gauze filter which fits inside the neck of the bottle.

A short piece of tubing from the delivery tube to a glass drip or drop counter.

A length of tubing connecting from the distal of the drop counter to the adaptor which fits the intravenous needle.

A tubing clip.

An adaptor and a stainless steel needle.

Tourniquet, preferably a sphygmomanometer cuff.

Local anæsthetic, hypodermic syringe and needles.

A disposable "giving" set is now in general use which is sterilized by autoclaving, used once and then discarded (Fig. 50). A nylon filter is incorporated in the drop-counter and a short piece of rubber tubing is included in the polythene delivery tubing near the needle adaptor so that drugs can be injected through the tubing if necessary.

Instruments for "cutting down" when it is not possible to enter the vein with a needle or if a continuous transfusion is required:

Scalpel.

One pair of fine toothed and one pair of fine non-toothed dissecting forceps.

One pair of fine pointed scissors.

Two "mosquito" fine artery forceps.

One aneurysm needle.

Thread, size 60, or catgut size 0, for tying in the cannula.

Two curved triangular needles and skin sutures.

Intravenous cannula, on fine polythene tubing.

Management of a Transfusion

Stored blood should be allowed to warm to room temperature before a transfusion is started, and the bottles should therefore be removed from the cold store about one hour before the transfusion is started.

Bottles containing blood should always be handled carefully to avoid shaking the contents.

When the transfusion has been satisfactorily started the prescribed rate of flow must be carefully maintained.

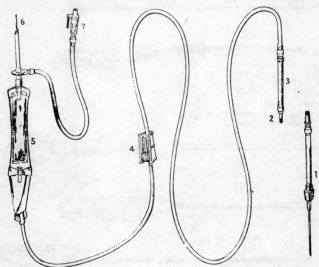

FIG. 50.—DISPOSABLE POLYTHENE "GIVING" SET.

(1) Needle with Luer fitting.
(2) Luer fitting mount.
(3) 2″ of rubber tubing for drugs to be added.
(4) Clip for regulating rate of flow through polythene tubing.
(5) Filter and drip.
(6) Needle to pierce bung of sterile infusion container.
(7) Air inlet filter to be hooked above fluid level in the container.

Forty drops per minute is the usual rate for a slow transfusion. Rapid transfusion may be required to replace blood loss and in such cases the transfusion of one or more bottles of blood may be given as quickly as it will flow into

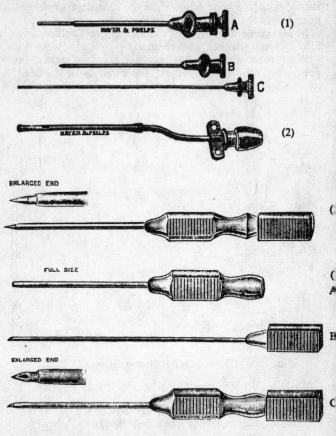

FIG. 51.—VARIOUS TYPES OF INTRAVENOUS CANNULÆ.

(1) Bateman's needle (for infants).
    A. Outer needle with stilette.
    B. Fine inner needle.
    C. Stilette.
(2) Hamilton Bailey's gold-plated cannula.
(3) Frankis Evans's intravenous needle.
(4) West Middlesex trocar and cannula.
    A. Outer cannula.
    B. Trocar.
    C. Cannula and trocar fitted together.

the vein. In cases of extreme urgency intra-arterial transfusion may be used.

As in many transfusions more than one bottle of blood will be needed, a fresh bottle must be obtained from the store in time to allow it to warm to room temperature before the bottle in use is empty. When the level of the blood in this bottle reaches a point just above the neck of the bottle the clip on the tubing above the drip connection is closed, the bottle is unhooked from the stand and placed on a trolley at the bedside on which the fresh bottle and a pair of sterile forceps have been set. The fresh bottle is opened using the sterile forceps to remove the washer, the rubber bung and tubes from the empty bottle are transferred to the new bottle. This operation must be carried out carefully, the tubing must not be allowed to touch the edge or the outside of either bottle during the process. The full bottle is then suspended from the hook of the transfusion stand, the clip on the rubber tubing is opened and the transfusion continued at the prescribed rate.

Difficulty in maintaining the flow of blood may be due to one of several causes. The vein may go into spasm. This may be overcome by gently warming the limb or by stroking along the vein above the injection site.

The tubing may become kinked or pressed upon and this possibility should always be borne in mind and careful inspection made.

The needle may become dislodged. An attempt may be made to alter the position of needle by gently lifting the mount to depress the point. This may be successful, but if the needle has punctured the wall of the vein the transfusion will have to be stopped and if necessary started again using another vein.

An air-lock may block the flow of blood from the bottle. This should not occur if due care is taken to expel all air from the delivery tubing before connecting it to the needle or cannula. If, however, an air-lock should be present the apparatus must be disconnected from the needle and blood allowed to run freely through the tubing before it is again connected to the intravenous needle.

Dangers that may arise during a Transfusion

The introduction of large volumes of blood, or any other fluid, into the blood-stream can give rise to cardiac and respiratory distress as a result of overloading the circulatory system. This danger is greatest when large quantities of fluid are rapidly introduced, but can occur with a slow transfusion particularly in elderly patients with a weakened heart muscle or chronic anæmia. Signs which should be watched for and reported to the medical officer immediately are: rising pulse rate, laboured breathing, cough, pain in the chest and œdema. A fluid intake and output chart should always be kept for a patient who is receiving parenteral fluid.

A severe reaction occurring soon after the transfusion has been started may be due to incompatibility of the blood and hæmolysis of the red cells. The symptoms are: shivering and rise of temperature, the patient may complain of severe pain in the lumbar region. The transfusion must be stopped at once. There is great danger of renal failure due to the blocking of the renal tubules by hæmolysed blood cells with subsequent suppression of urine and uræmia.

Pyrexial reaction due to the introduction of foreign protein into the blood can also give rise to rigors, fever and an increased pulse rate. The rate of the transfusion should be slowed, or the transfusion may have to be stopped.

Thrombosis of the vein is not uncommon. It may be limited in extent and cause little trouble, but if extensive there is considerable pain in the limb and there may be a rise in the patient's temperature. The transfusion may have to be discontinued and a hot application may be ordered for the relief of pain.

A hæmatoma may form at the site of the transfusion, this results from the needle becoming dislodged from the vein and the blood is then extravasated into the surrounding tissues. The transfusion must be stopped and the limb elevated. An injection of hyalase may be given into the swollen area. There is some danger when the swelling occurs on the anterior aspect of the forearm and elbow that the arteries supplying the forearm may be compressed and careful watch should be kept on the radial pulse and also on the fingers for blueness and coldness.

Sepsis may occur at the site of the infusion. This is more liable to occur when a cannula is tied into the vein than with the use of an intravenous needle.

Air embolism is a rare occurrence but one which must be borne in mind. It is prevented by making sure that air is entirely expelled from the tubing before the transfusion is started and by taking care that the bottle is not allowed to run dry. The patient may complain of a variety of sensory disturbances—*e.g.* tingling in the fingers, and may collapse. The immediate treatment is to lower the patient's head.

Subcutaneous Infusion of Saline. The method is more commonly used for children than adults, and an infant of six months may be expected to absorb about 2 fl. oz., 60 ml., of fluid from each site. For older patients up to 300 ml. may be given.

Requirements:

Y-shaped glass connection.

Bottle of sterile saline solution with tubing and drop counter.

Two pieces of rubber tubing to fit the arms of the connection.

Two needles.

1-ml. syringe.

Ampoules of hyaluronidase (Hyalase) and sterile distilled water.

Two small bulldog clips.

Sterile swabs and towels.

Ether or cetrimide for cleaning the skin.

Small gauze dressing.

Adhesive strapping or collodion.

Scissors and dissecting forceps.

Instrument forceps in jar.

Receptacle for soiled swabs.

The needles are attached to the ends of the rubber tubing. The skin of the area chosen is cleaned. Saline, is allowed to run through the apparatus to expel the air. The tubing is then clipped. A fold of subcutaneous tissue (usually the axilla or the area below the breasts is chosen) is picked up with the left hand and with the right one of the needles is inserted into the subcutaneous tissue in an upward direction. The second needle is inserted into the other side. The clip is removed and the fluid allowed to run in slowly.

The bacterial ferment hyaluronidase (Hyalase) is often used to promote the absorption of fluid. When the flow of saline has been started, 0·5 ml. of Hyalase is injected through each of the two pieces of tubing connected to the subcutaneous needles.

When a subcutaneous infusion is given by the drip method the needles, once they have been inserted, may be kept in place by two small pieces of adhesive strapping. A piece of wool or gamgee tissue should cover the area.

21

Gastric Lavage and Aspiration

WASHING out the stomach is a procedure that may be ordered in cases of pyloric stenosis, in intestinal obstruction immediately before operation and in the treatment for poisoning when the poison has been swallowed, particularly in cases of narcotic poisoning or acute alcoholic poisoning. A stomach wash-out may be given in the treatment of poisoning by a corrosive or caustic substance after the poison has been neutralized.

Requirements:

> Jacques's œsophageal catheter, for an adult sizes 18 to 20, for a child sizes 8 to 14 and for an infant a soft rubber catheter, size 8.
>
> A glass connection.
>
> A length of rubber tubing (3 to 4 feet).
>
> A large glass funnel.
>
> Large jug containing the solution for the wash-out, *e.g.* tap water, sodium bicarbonate 1 drachm to water 1 pint, or normal saline 6 pints, which should be prepared at a temperature of 100° F.
>
> A pint measure.
>
> A large pail to receive the wash-out.
>
> A receiver for tube after use.
>
> A mouth wash and a few small squares of old linen.
>
> A lubricant, such as glycerin or butter, may be required.
>
> A mackintosh to protect the bedclothes and a mackintosh cape to protect the patient's gown.
>
> A gag will be required if the patient is unconscious.

Method. The apparatus should be placed in a bowl of hot water. The pail stands on the floor at the bedside and should be placed on newspaper to protect the floor. If the patient is conscious and able to co-operate, the usual position is sitting upright leaning slightly forward; if he is unconscious, the usual procedure is to have him prone, with the head over the edge of the bed or couch, or else on his back with the head lower than the body.

The tube should be marked at 16 and 18 inches.

The tube is easier to swallow if it has been chilled on ice before use.

The tube should be passed over the tongue slightly to one side of the midline towards the pharynx and the patient, if conscious, is directed to swallow, the tube peing pushed along as he does so. He should be allowed time to breathe and directed to take a fairly big breath between swallowing. The average distance from the lips to the cardiac orifice of the stomach is 16 inches, so that when 18 inches of the tube have been swallowed it is safely in the stomach.

The pint measure is filled with solution from the large jug and about 1 pint is allowed to flow in. When the funnel is almost empty, it should be inverted over the pail and the fluid syphoned back. The process is repeated until the fluid is returned clear or until the prescribed amount of the solution has been used.

The tube should then be tightly compressed and with-drawn quickly. The patient should be given the mouth wash and the pieces of old linen to wipe his mouth. The contents of the pail should be measured and saved for inspection.

Several gallons of fluid may be needed to wash out the stomach in cases of poisoning. If unconscious the patient is placed in either the prone or Trendelenburg's position to prevent fluid running into the air passages. The lavage in cases of poisoning is performed by the doctor.

Aspiration of stomach contents for diagnostic purposes or to empty the stomach as in acute gastric dilatation or paralytic ileus is usually carried out by means of a Ryle's tube, a small œsophageal catheter (size 6) or a Miller-Abbot's tube passed through the nose and left in position. The lubricated tube is passed along the floor of the nose until it reaches the pharynx. The patient may then be given sips of water and the tube is pushed on by the operator while the movements of swallowing are taking place. The stomach contents are aspirated by a syringe attached to the end of the tube or by continuous suction using a siphonage apparatus. A simple siphonage apparatus may be set up if continuous suction is required using a large bottle containing water which is suspended neck downwards, about three feet above the level of the patient's body. The bottle is closed with a two-hole rubber bung through which pass one short

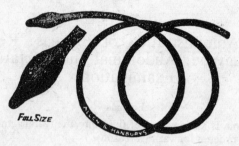

Fig. 52.—Ryle's Tube.

and one long piece of glass tubing. The short tube is connected by a length of rubber tubing to a similar bottle standing on the floor and the rate of flow of water from the upper to the lower bottle is controlled by a screw tubing clip. The longer piece of glass tubing which projects beyond the water level in the suspended bottle is connected to the Ryle's or Miller-Abbott's tube.

22

The Administration of Enemas: Rectal Lavage: Abdominal and Rectal Examinations

Enemas

AN enema is an injection of fluid into the rectum and this may be ordered for various reasons:

(1) To empty the bowel of fæces.
(2) To relieve distension due to flatus.
(3) To introduce drugs or fluids.
(4) For diagnostic purposes.

Apparatus. For large quantities such as are used for cleansing the bowel, a douche can, a piece of rubber tubing about 24 inches long, a glass connection and a rubber rectal tube or catheter, size 14 or 16, are required. A Higginson's syringe with a rubber rectal tube attached is occasionally used and in this case the solution to be injected is placed in a bowl. For small quantities a glass funnel or the barrel of a glass syringe is connected to a rubber catheter (size 8). The same apparatus is usually used for giving an enema to a child.

Important Points to be observed in giving an Enema. The rectum is not a straight tube, it curves backwards, following the contour of the coccyx and the sacrum. The rectal tube should be passed first forward and upward, through the anal canal, which is approximately two inches in length, into the lower end of the rectum.

The flow of the fluid will be helped if the patient lies on her left side, or, if on her back, has the pelvis raised during the administration of the enema. The douche can should be raised about 12 inches above the level of the patient's body.

The length of the rectum is about 6 inches, and if more

than 4 to 6 inches of the tube is passed it is liable to kink or to become coiled upon itself. This is uncomfortable for the patient and also obstructs the flow of the enema fluid.

No force should be used in passing a rectal tube. If the anal sphincter is tightly closed or the patient has hæmorrhoids, which make the part very sensitive, it may be necessary to dilate the sphincter before passing the tube, using the finger protected by a rubber glove or finger stall lubricated with petroleum jelly. The tube should be well lubricated and air expelled by allowing the fluid to run through, before inserting it.

The tube should be inserted about 4 inches into the rectum, so that it is well gripped by the anal sphincter, and a brief pause should follow the insertion before allowing the fluid to flow. To ensure that the fluid flows right round to the cæcum, when this is required for cleansing or for treatment, it should not be injected too quickly and the pelvis should be raised (if this is not possible, the foot of the bed may be raised).

The enema must be given at the right temperature, usually 100° F. If it is too hot or too cold, the fluid will be returned at once and the patient is caused unnecessary discomfort.

A report of the result of the enema should always be made, and, if necessary the result saved for inspection. If obstruction is suspected it is important to note the passage of flatus.

The procedure should always be simply explained to the patient before beginning the treatment. A very ill patient or a patient who has been given an enema for the relief of distension, when it is important to note if flatus is passed, should not be left until the bed-pan has been removed.

It is usual to protect the bed with a warmed mackintosh, which may be covered with a cotton square or a piece of cellulose. After giving the enema, the rectal catheter should be disconnected and placed in a receiver so that it does not soil anything else. It should be flushed through with cold water, washed well with warm soapy water to remove the grease and boiled for five minutes.

Complications that may result from giving an enema are:

(1) Faintness and collapse, due to the distension of the rectum with fluid.

(2) An enema rash. If the patient states that on a previous occasion a rash followed the giving of a soap enema, this should be reported.

(3) Possible perforation of the rectal wall if a rigid nozzle is used.

1. **Cleansing Enemas.**—*Water*. A suitable quantity of warm water injected into the bowel will distend the rectum, wash out the lower bowel and produce an evacuant action. Water is as effective and less irritating than the traditional soap and water enema. The quantity required will vary from a few ounces for a young child to 1 to 3 pints for an adult.

Soap and Water. From 1 to 3 pints of the solution will be required for an adult.

A soap solution ready made up is often used in hospital, and the enema is prepared by adding the directed quantity of the soap solution to hot water. Green soft soap one ounce to one pint of water may be used, and a piece about the size of a large walnut will be required for every pint of water. The soap should be well beaten into the water and the solution strained before use.

Recently attention has been drawn to the fact that the injection of large quantities of water or of soap and water into the bowel can be a dangerous process as these fluids are rapidly absorbed from the colon into the blood stream and may bring about a serious change in the concentration of electrolytes in the blood. The symptoms produced are due to what is known as "water intoxication" and include nausea, vomiting and drowsiness which may proceed to a state of coma and convulsions; the patient's breathing may become rapid and irregular. The danger is greatest in young children and when repeated enemas are given. It is important that the nurse should be aware of this danger and that she should appreciate the importance of accurate measurement of the fluid injected and the fluid returned when administering enemas or any form of bowel wash-out. The sodium phosphate enema described below is considerably safer from this point of view in that only a small quantity of fluid is injected.

Sodium Phosphate Enema. Recently the use of mixed sodium phosphates dissolved in a small quantity of water as an evacuant enema has been adopted in hospital practice and in home nursing. A solution of sodium dihydrogen phosphate 14 grammes and disodium hydrogen phosphate 4 grammes in 120 ml. of water is equally, if not more effective than a soap and water enema and causes the patient less discomfort. Disposable plastic units with a plastic or rubber injection tube are available. Very little is needed for the preparation and administration of the enema; the apparatus is used once only so that the task of cleaning and boiling equipment after use is eliminated.

Glycerin. A small quantity (from 1 to 3 fluid ounces) of glycerin may be mixed with an equal amount of warm water and given with a catheter and funnel. A special glass and vulcanite syringe may be used if the glycerin is given undiluted, a soft rubber catheter should be attached to the hard vulcanite nozzle of the syringe. Suppositories of glycerin and gelatin have largely replaced the glycerin enema. The glycerin enema or suppository is useful in producing an action of the bowels with little disturbance of the patient, glycerin also has the effect of softening hard masses of fæces in the rectum. *90. - 950;-*

Olive Oil. Warm olive oil may be ordered to soften the fæces after operations on the rectum or perineum (when it is necessary to ensure that no hard masses be passed), or in cases of impacted fæces; 4 to 10 oz. of warm olive oil is slowly injected with a catheter and funnel. The patient should retain this for at least half an hour, and the treatment is completed by giving a soap-and-water enema if ordered.

2. **Enemas for the Relief of Distension.**—*Ox-bile Enema* (*Enema Fellis Bovini*). 2 to 4 drachms of fresh ox-bile or 15 gr. of ox-bile extract with ½ pint of soap and water. If dried ox-bile is used it is prepared by adding 4 oz. of boiling water and when the solution has cooled it is added to 6 oz. of soap and water solution. *paralytic Ileus = brewron pertesd*

Turpentine Enema (*Enema Terebinthinæ*). 120 to 480 minims of turpentine, 1 pint of soap and water.

The oil of turpentine is irritating and liable to burn the tissues if floating in globules in the mixture. It is therefore commonly made into an emulsion with a mucilaginous substance or with olive oil. To prevent burning of the anal region the area should first be protected with an application of petroleum jelly.

Method 1. Beat the turpentine with olive oil using 1 fl. oz. of oil for every 60 minims of turpentine, make the total volume up to 1 pint with soap solution, beating well, and give at a temperature of 100° F. Follow with the remainder of the pint of soap and water.

Method 2. Add the turpentine to 4 oz. of starch mucilage and give this, following with ½ to 1 pint of soap and water.

Method 3. Make 1 pint of soap and water solution with boiling water, add the turpentine slowly, drop by drop, beating well all the time, until the required amount has been added and the temperature of the mixture has cooled to 100° F.

Passing a Flatus Tube for the Relief of Distension.

Requirements:

    A rubber rectal tube. This tube has thick walls and the eye is at the end. In this respect it differs from a catheter which has a lateral eye.

    A glass connection attaching the rectal tube to a length of rubber tubing with a glass funnel at other end.

    A bowl of water.

    Petroleum jelly, or other lubricant and swabs.

    A receiver for soiled swabs.

    A mackintosh square and pad to protect the bed.

The tube is lubricated and passed into the rectum for about 2 inches. The funnel is placed under the surface of the water in the bowl which is placed at the bedside. Another method is to use a rectal tube without the length of rubber tubing attached and to place a receiver under the opening of the tube. A layer of cellulose may be placed under and another layer over the part of the tube resting in the receiver. The advantage of attaching the tube to a funnel placed in a bowl of water is that the bubbles of gas can be readily seen as they escape from the funnel.

3. Enemas used to introduce drugs for their general or local effect.—*Magnesium Sulphate Enema.* Magnesium sulphate solution given as an enema attracts fluid from the tissues into the bowel. It may be ordered as an evacuant and also in cases of raised intracranial tension in order to relieve the tension by causing dehydration of the tissues. For this purpose 6 to 8 fl. ozs. of a 50 per cent. solution of magnesium sulphate may be given twice a day for several days.

Starch and Opium Enema. A starch mucilage usually with the addition of tincture of opium may be ordered for the relief of diarrhœa. A starch and opium enema consists of 15 to 30 minims of tincture of opium as ordered, 2 to 4 oz. of starch mucilage.

1 oz. of the starch mucilage should be injected slowly at body temperature, using a No. 8 catheter and a small funnel or barrel of a glass syringe, then the ordered amount of opium is given, followed by a sufficient amount of the mucilage to clear the opium from the funnel and tubing.

To make the mucilage take a dessertspoonful of powdered starch and sufficient cold water to make a stiff paste. Add sufficient boiling water to make a fluid which will be thin enough to run through the enema apparatus when cooled to 100° F.

An alternative method is to take 1 level dessertspoonful of starch, mixing this to a smooth thin paste with 5 oz. of cold water. The mixture is brought to the boil and boiled for 2 minutes. One teaspoonful of cold water is added and the mucilage is allowed to cool.

Cortisone Enema. Hydrocortisone in normal saline may be ordered as a retention enema in the treatment of ulcerative colitis. 100 mg. of hydrocortisone hemi-succinate is mixed with about 120 ml. of normal saline. The enema is given at body heat using a rubber catheter and a small funnel. The administration should take 20 to 30 minutes.

Diagnostic Enema. The barium sulphate emulsion for use in barium enema X-ray examinations is usually made up in the dispensary in the form of a barium suspension.

The following prescription is one in use:

Barium sulphate ..	..	..	.. 40 oz.
Tragacanth powder	..	..	60 grains
Water ..	..	..	To 80 fluid oz.

This is to be diluted with an equal quantity of water for use. The water added to the emulsion should be hot enough to bring the mixture to body temperature.

The colon and rectum should be empty before the barium enema is administered, an aperient is usually ordered twenty-four hours beforehand and a rectal wash-out given about four hours before the X-ray examination. The preparation used in some diagnostic X-ray departments may

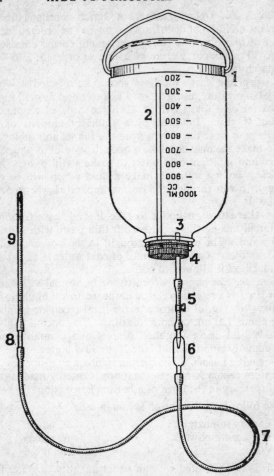

FIG. 53.—APPARATUS FOR "CONTINUOUS DRIP" ENEMA.
1. Metal band and handle for suspension.
2. Metal tube acting as an air inlet.
3. Metal outlet tube.
4. Black rubber bung.
5. Short piece of rubber tubing and screw clip.
6. Drop counter.
7. Length of rubber tubing.
8. Glass connection.
9. Rubber catheter.

vary from that described and exact instructions should always be obtained.

Retention Enemas as a Means of administering Fluid. Rectal administration of normal saline solution or of water is a method of supplementing the fluid intake when the patient for any reason is unable to take sufficient fluid by mouth. 5 or 10 per cent. glucose may be added.

If the patient is to retain and absorb the fluid satisfactorily the following points must receive attention:

(1) The rectum and the bladder must be empty.

(2) The fluid must be injected slowly.

Method 1. The required amount of tap water or saline and glucose solution, usually not more than 10 oz., is run in slowly, using a No. 8 rubber catheter and a small funnel or the barrel of a glass syringe.

In order to have complete control over the rate of flow the funnel should be held at a level only slightly above that of the patient's body. The rate of flow must be slow and even.

10 oz. of fluid should take at least ten minutes to give. The patient should be left undisturbed for half an hour after the injection.

This method may also be used for the injection of basal anæsthetics or narcotics such as paraldehyde and bromethol.

Method 2 ("*Continuous Drip*"). A glass bottle is required, fitted with a rubber bung with two holes.

A short glass tube fixed in one hole is connected to a piece of rubber tubing with a screw-clip. A further piece of rubber tubing, an ordinary glass connection, and a No. 7 or 8 rubber catheter are required.

A second glass tube long enough to reach to the far end of the bottle passes through the second hole in the bung, this acts as an airway.

The fluid is allowed to run through the tubing to expel the air, and the tubing is then clipped and the container suspended at the bedside neck downwards. The tubing clip is regulated to give the required rate of flow (about 1 drop per second). Several pints of fluid may be slowly introduced by this method.

The nurse should see that the steady rate of flow is maintained and should also make sure from time to time that the patient is retaining the fluid.

10*

Rectal and Colonic Lavage

This treatment may be ordered in the preparation of a patient for examination by sigmoidoscopy or for a barium enema examination. (Dulcolax tablets and suppositories may replace lavage, particularly for out-patients.)

Requirements:

A rubber catheter, size 14, [12] or rectal tube.

A length of rubber tubing.

A tubing clip.

A glass connection to fit the rubber tubing and the catheter.

Lubricant and swabs.

A large jug containing the washout fluid, usually water or normal saline. Six pints or more may be needed.

An irrigating can, or a large funnel and a pint measure jug.

A pail to receive returned fluid or a large bed-pan.

Receiver for soiled swabs and catheter.

The water or lotion should be prepared at a temperature of 105° F. and used at a temperature of 100° F.

The catheter is lubricated, fluid is poured into the irrigating can and allowed to run through the apparatus to expel air and the tubing is then clamped with the tubing clip. If a funnel is used in place of the irrigating can it is filled from the pint measure jug. *[a pint at a time.]*

The patient lies on his left side with the knees flexed and the catheter is passed into the rectum for a distance of about three inches. The clip is released and fluid allowed to flow, it should run in slowly at first as sudden distension of the rectum may cause the patient to return the fluid. When one pint has been given the patient should, if possible turn into the "knee-chest" position while a further pint is allowed to run in steadily, then he assumes the right lateral position while the third pint is given. The tubing is then clipped, the catheter removed and the patient placed on the bed-pan and allowed to return the wash-out fluid.

[colonic] An alternative method is to run in about half a pint of fluid using a large funnel and then to siphon it back by inverting the funnel over a pail. The process is repeated until the fluid returns clear.

[colonic requires more quantities, raise end of bed.]

Accurate measurement of the fluid given and the fluid returned must always be made. *to prevent retention of fluid*

Abdominal Examination

The bed should be screened and nearby windows closed. The patient should lie on her back with the knees slightly flexed and one pillow under the head and shoulders. The bedclothes should be turned down to the thighs and the patient left covered with the sheet. The nightgown should be folded up to the breasts and a small blanket or shawl arranged to cover the chest. When the doctor is ready to make the examination the nurse should turn down the sheet and arrange the chest blanket so that the area from the breasts to the pubes is bare. During the examination the nurse should stand at the left-hand side of the bed at the head end. Requirements for rectal examination should be at hand.

Rectal Examination

Requirements:

A right-hand rubber glove or finger stall.
Glove powder.
Lubricant.
Swabs.
Receiver.
A rectal speculum and a hand lamp may be needed.

The patient should, if possible lie in the left lateral position with the buttocks brought to the edge of the bed and the knees flexed.

The gown should be folded up over the chest; a blanket is arranged to cover the chest and the buttocks are covered by a sheet only During the examination the nurse should stand at the right-hand side of the bed.

Examination by Sigmoidoscopy

This examination is carried out in the theatre. It is important that the rectum should be emptied of fæces and also of any fluid given as an enema or rectal wash-out.

The actual preparation will vary according to the wish of the surgeon, but the following may be taken as a guide:

Thirty-six hours before the examination the patient is given an aperient.

Twelve hours before the examination the patient is given a soap-and-water enema or a rectal wash-out with plain warm water. The nurse should measure all fluid injected and the fluid returned.

Following this preparation a dose of tincture of opium may be ordered to allay further bowel movement.

23

Catheterization, Irrigation and Drainage of the Urinary Bladder

Catheterization

CATHETERIZATION of the urinary bladder may be required to relieve distension of the bladder when the patient is unable to pass urine, to empty the bladder before an operation on the pelvic organs or to obtain a specimen of urine for examination.

Varieties of Catheters

(1) *Soft Rubber.* These are in sizes from 1 to 20, English gauge. The size most often required for catheterization is 8.

(2) *Elastic Gum.* In the same sizes as the rubber catheters. French catheters, however, are numbered from 1 to 30. The elastic gum catheter may be straight with a bulbous or cylindrical end, or may be angled or "elbowed" near the eye. In the latter case it is known as a coudé catheter. If it has two bends it is a bicoudé catheter. Silk web catheters are semi-stiff, similar to the elastic gum ones, but are usually grey or white, while the elastic gum catheters are brown or black. Silk catheters are provided with a wire stilette.

(3) *Glass Catheters.* Used for female patients only.

(4) *Metal Catheters.* These are made in both the male and female patterns. Metal female catheters may be used in midwifery practice.

Catheterization of a Male Patient. The doctor will select the catheters, but if there are no special orders the nurse should sterilize rubber and elastic gum catheters, sizes 7 and 8.

Requirements:

Sterile catheters in a sterile tray dry or in cold sterile water, normal saline or boracic lotion.

A lubricant, such as sterile glycerin or liquid paraffin.
Sterile towels and swabs.
Bowl of warm lotion for swabbing, *e.g.* Hibitane 0·1 per
cent., Bradosol 1 in 2,000 solution.
Large receiver for urine.
Mackintosh.
Receiver for dirty swabs.
(If a "clean" specimen for examination is required, a
sterile screw-top bottle to receive the urine must be
provided.)

The bed is screened and the bedclothes arranged so that
they can be easily turned down over the thighs, leaving the
abdomen and chest covered with a blanket.

After the trolley is brought to the bedside the nurse is
not usually required to give any further assistance.

If the catheter is to be tied in, the following should also
be provided:

Tape.
Adhesive strapping.
A pair of scissors.

If urethral bougies are to be passed these are sterilized in
the same way as catheters.   The same trolley should be set
as for catheterization.

Catheterization of a Female Patient

Requirements:

Two sterilized catheters in a sterile bowl or dish.
A bowl of lotion for swabbing.
Sterile swabs and towels.
Mackintosh.
Large receiver for urine.
Receiver for dirty swabs.
A hand lamp.
A lubricant is not as a rule required.
(When a sterile specimen is required a sterile screw-top
bottle should be provided, and all traces of antiseptics
should be removed by swabbing with sterile water.)

The bed should be screened and the bedclothes turned
down from the patient's knees, leaving her covered with a
blanket.   A warmed mackintosh is placed under the patient's
thighs and buttocks and a receiver or a porringer between
her legs.   The hand lamp should be adjusted so that it gives

a good light; it is absolutely essential that the nurse should be able to obtain a clear view of the area when swabbing the external genitals and when actually passing the catheter.

The nurse then prepares her hands by washing and drying them on a clean towel. When she returns to the bedside she turns back the covering blanket with her elbow, or asks an assistant to do this for her.

Using swabs well moistened with the antiseptic lotion she swabs the external genital region beginning with the labia majora, then swabbing the labia minora and lastly the area around the urethral orifice. Each swab should be used once only and the direction of swabbing should be from the anterior aspect of the vulva towards the posterior margin. The nurse should then wash her hands once more and arrange the sterile towels to cover the patient's thighs. The catheter should be picked up in the right hand, the first finger and thumb of the left hand being used to separate the labia. The urethral orifice should be clearly seen and a good light is essential, the opening is situated immediately in front of the vaginal orifice and at the base of the triangular area known as the vestibule. A glass or metal catheter may be held sufficiently far from the tip to ensure that the section handled does not enter the urethra, this is more difficult with a soft rubber catheter and sterile forceps or piece of sterile gauze may be used to avoid direct handling of the catheter. The tip of the catheter is passed into the urethral orifice and then the instrument is pushed on in an upward and backward direction for about two inches, leaving the open end in the receiver between the patient's thighs. If the catheter should accidentally touch any adjacent part before it is safely inserted in the urethra it should be discarded as probably contaminated and the second sterile catheter should then be used.

If a catheter specimen is required for laboratory examination it is collected in a sterile screw-top glass bottle.

When urine ceases to flow the nurse should make gentle pressure over the pubes and withdraw the catheter for about half an inch, when she feels sure that the bladder is empty the catheter is withdrawn and placed in the receiver provided. The porringer is removed, the vulva dried and the bed remade. The amount of urine withdrawn should be measured and a specimen saved if required.

Catheterization is a procedure that should be carried out with the utmost care with regard to the sterilization of the catheters, the cleansing of the vulva beforehand and the skilful manipulation of the catheter. Infection of the urinary tract can occur very readily and may be very serious: Patients who are being regularly catheterized are often given a urinary antiseptic, such as potassium or sodium citrate or one of the sulphonamide drugs.

Irrigation of the Bladder

Requirements: As for catheterization, with the following additions:

A glass connection which will fit the end of the catheter.
3 to 4 feet of rubber tubing to fit the connection.
A glass funnel.
A clip.
A lotion thermometer.
A jug containing the sterile lotion (2 or more pints).
A bowl to receive the returned lotion.

The glass connection tubing and funnel must all be sterilized. Usually normal saline solution or sterile water is used: the temperature of the lotion should be 100° F. The catheter should first be passed and the bladder emptied. The tubing should be filled with the lotion and clipped; it is then attached by the glass connection to the catheter. The funnel should be filled with lotion and raised about 1 foot above the level of the patient's body so that the fluid flows gently into the bladder. When the lotion begins to rise back into the funnel this indicates that the bladder is full. The fluid should be siphoned back by lowering the funnel and inverting it over the bowl provided and the amount measured, so that the capacity of the bladder is known. About 1 fluid ounce less than this quantity is then allowed to flow in and siphoned back, continuing until the return fluid is clear

Bladder irrigation is most commonly ordered for the treatment of cystitis, and in this condition the bladder may only hold 1 or 2 fl. oz.; but as the condition improves and the inflammation of the bladder subsides its capacity increases and a note should be made of the amount every time the treatment is carried out.

For washing out the bladder in a male patient a metal

bladder syringe is used and the solution injected through the catheter. The syringe is disconnected and the fluid allowed to run back into a large receiver placed between the patient's thighs. The catheter may be left in position after the treatment and the end closed with a spigot.

Tidal drainage (Fig. 54). In some forms of residual infection of the bladder, especially those associated with

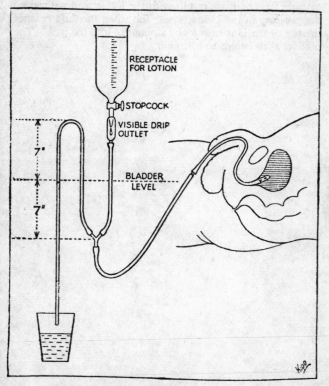

FIG. 54.—TIDAL DRAINAGE.

paraplegia, a combination of drainage and irrigation may be carried out. A large receptacle for the irrigating lotion is connected to a drip outlet which in turn is joined by a piece of rubber tubing to one arm of a Y-shaped glass connection. The stem of this connection is attached to a catheter in the patient's bladder, the remaining arm to a length of rubber tubing which is looped to form a U-shaped manometer fourteen inches high with the centre at the level of the patient's bladder. The end of this long piece of tubing opens into a pail on the floor which collects the fluid. The lotion is allowed to drip slowly into the bladder via the catheter; as the bladder fills with the lotion and with urine the pressure in the U loop rises, and when the fluid reaches the top of the U it empties by siphonage into the pail. The bladder then begins to fill again.

24

Vaginal Examination, Douching, Vulval Toilet: Vaginal Pessaries

Vaginal Examination

THE patient may be examined in bed or in the theatre, when an anæsthetic may be given.

Positions for Gynæcological Examinations

Dorsal. As described for abdominal examination.

Left Lateral. As described for rectal examination.

Semi-lateral or Sims's Position. The patient lies on her left side with the buttocks brought to the side of the bed and the upper leg rather more flexed than the under one. The head and chest should lie prone on the bed with one small pillow. The left arm hangs over the edge of the bed and the right arm is brought up alongside the pillow.

The Upright Position. The patient stands at the side of a chair with one foot resting on the rung and steadying herself with one hand on the back of the chair. This position is sometimes required when an examination is made for prolapse.

Lithotomy Position. The patient lies on her back with the knees flexed and the thighs raised and separated. The buttocks are brought to the edge of the couch, the legs are supported in stirrups and the foot end of the examination couch is dropped.

Requirements for vaginal examination:

Right-hand rubber gloves.

Receptacles for soiled swabs and for used instruments.

If the patient is being examined on account of pregnancy or abortion sterile gloves are required.

A bowl of lotion—*e.g.* Hibitane 0·1 per cent. Cetrimide 1 per cent. solution.

Swabs.

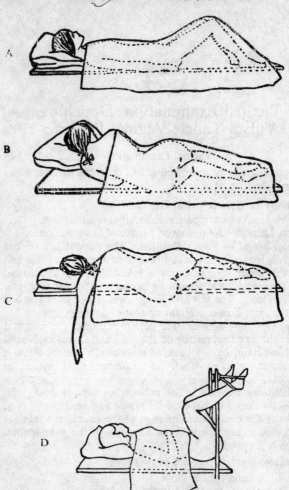

FIG. 55.—GYNÆCOLOGICAL POSITIONS.

A.—Dorsal Position.
B.—Left Lateral Position.
C.—Sims's Position.
D.—Lithotomy Position.

Swab-holding forceps.

Vaginal specula: Sims's duckbill, Ferguson's and bi-
valve patterns.

If a smear of discharge from the cervix is required the
following requirements should be prepared:

Ferguson's speculum.

Vulsellum forceps.

Swabs and a swab-holder.

A platinum wire loop, or sterile throat swabs.

Microscope slides.

A spirit lamp.

Labels.

Requirements for rectal examination should be provided.

Preparation of the Patient

The rectum should be empty and an aperient may be
ordered the day before the examination. The patient
should empty the bladder shortly beforehand, but, as the
gynæcologist may wish to examine the urethral meatus for
the presence of any discharge, she should not do so
immediately before presenting herself to the doctor as the
passing of urine will wash away any urethral discharge.
Out-patients should be instructed to remove all top clothing
and corsets and to come to the examination room wearing
a vest, stockings, slippers and a dressing gown.

Vaginal Douching

Vaginal douching is usually carried out for cleansing
purposes, *i.e.* in cases of vaginal discharge, before operations
on the female genital tract and may be ordered as a routine
cleansing measure for patients wearing vaginal pessaries.
Hot douching at a temperature of 115°–120° F. may be used
in arresting uterine hæmorrhage and for the treatment of
pelvic inflammation although in the former case it is not very
effective and in the latter case the advent of chemotherapeutic drugs has resulted in local treatment being less
frequently ordered than formerly.

Requirements:

A douche can.

Long piece of rubber tubing.

Douche nozzle, rubber or glass, or a rubber catheter,
size 10.

Clip.

Douche lotion.

Antiseptic lotion for swabbing—*e.g.* Hibitane 1 per cent.

Sterile swabs and pads.

Bowl for soiled swabs.

Douche pan.

The douche can, tubing nozzle or catheter are sterilized and placed in a sterile bowl.

The lotion for douching is prepared as ordered and at a temperature of 105° F. As a general rule only mild lotions are used, except in cases of purulent discharge. Normal saline solution, hypertonic saline sterile water flavine 1 in 1,000 solution and 1 per cent. lactic acid are examples of solutions which may be ordered.

At least 3 pints of lotion will be required. When it has been prepared and the temperature tested it should be poured into the douche can and the tubing clipped. The can should be hung about 2 feet above the level of the patient's body.

The patient lies on her back on the douche pan (the "perfection" type of bed-pan is very often used). The sheet under the douche pan should be protected by a mackintosh.

Before the nurse washes her hands the bedclothes should be so arranged that the patient's thighs and legs are covered by a blanket and sheet while her chest and abdomen are covered by a folded blanket. When the nurse returns from washing her hands and drying them on a clean towel she pushes the lower half of the divided bedclothes down using her elbow. Taking a swab in her right hand she first swabs the labia majora with the antiseptic lotion provided and then parting the labia with the first finger and thumb of her left hand she swabs the labia minora and the area of the vaginal orifice. The swabbing should be carried out from above downwards and each swab should be used once only. The tubing clip is released allowing the lotion to flow through the apparatus. The douche nozzle or catheter is then inserted gently upwards and backwards into the vagina for about 3 inches.

When the douche is completed the patient should sit up on the douche pan for a few moments to allow the fluid to drain out of the vagina. The vulva is then dried with sterile swabs and a sterile pad applied.

A glass douche nozzle should always be carefully inspected before use to make sure that it is not cracked or chipped. In all cases where stitches have been inserted into the perineum or vagina it is safer to use a rubber catheter.

Vulval Toilet

In obstetric cases and in cases where the vulval or perineal area has been sutured, careful vulval toilet is necessary for the comfort of the patient and also in order to prevent infection of the sutured area.

1. Vulval Swabbing and Dressing of Sutures

Requirements:

Sterile kidney dish.

Sterile bowl containing warm antiseptic lotion such as domiphen bromide (Bradosol) 1 in 2,000 solution or plain water.

Sterile bowl containing sterile swabs, gauze vulval pads, two pairs of dressing forceps.

Receptacle for soiled swabs and dressings.

First of all the patient's groins and the inner aspect of the thighs should be washed with soap and water and dried. The nurse should then wash and dry her hands. Taking a well moistened swab in her left hand she swabs the external aspect of the labia then, discarding that swab, she parts the labia with her left hand and with her right hand swabs the inner aspect of each labium, using one swab for each side. Next the area of the vestibule and the vaginal orifice is swabbed. The area should then be carefully dried and the vulval pad applied. The patient is then asked to bring her thighs together and to turn on her side. The vulval pad is folded back exposing the perineal area

The suture area is dried with a sterile swab held in forceps and the antiseptic paint or powder is applied. The sutures are then covered with gauze, taking care to wrap the long ends of the sutures in the gauze so that they do not catch in the vulval pad when the patient moves. The vulval pad is brought down to cover the dressing and the pad is kept in place with a T bandage.

2. **"Jug" Douching.** For this procedure a two-pint jug containing warm antiseptic lotion or warm water and a large

receiver or douche pan will be required, in addition to the times listed above.

Some of the lotion is first poured over the vulva and then the nurse separates the labia with her left hand and continues pouring the remainder of the lotion so that the flow of antiseptic cleanses the labia minora and vaginal orifice. On completion of the douching, the area is carefully dried with swabs and sterile vulval pad applied. If sutures have to be dressed the patient now turns on her side and this procedure is carried out as described above.

Vaginal Pessaries

A pessary is an instrument introduced into the vagina usually in order to afford support in the case of a prolapsed uterus. Pessaries are made of vulcanite, perspex or coils of watch spring covered with rubber. Pessaries used in the treatment of uterine prolapse may be ring shaped or, if the vaginal walls and perineum are too lax to allow the ring to remain in position a circular cup with a stem, Napier's pessary, is inserted. The cup supports the cervix and the stem is attached by four tapes to a band round the patient's waist. The use of pessaries in the treatment of genital prolapse is now comparatively rare, since the majority of patients can be far more satisfactorily treated by operative measures. The nurse may be required to change a ring pessary.

Insertion of a Ring Pessary

Requirements:

> Sterilized introducer or clip forceps and a length of tape.
> Sterilized pessary, vulcanite, watch spring or plastic.
> Swabs in lotion—Bradosol 1 in 2,000 solution.
> Sterile lubricant.
> Sterile gloves.
> Mackintosh.
> Receptacle for soiled swabs.
> Receiver for discarded gloves.
> A good light is essential and an adjustable standard or hand lamp may be needed.

The patient is placed in the left lateral position and a mackintosh is arranged to protect the bed or couch. Before the pessary is inserted the nurse should swab the vulva and then after washing her hands again puts on the sterilized gloves. Taking the pessary in her right hand she dips it in the lubricant. The nurse's left hand is used to separate the labia. The ring is then inserted into the vagina with the posterior rim along the length of the orifice gradually turning it over directing it upwards and backwards until one side of the rim of the ring is in the posterior fornix and the cervix can be felt in the centre of the ring. The anterior rim is then pushed up above the symphysis pubis. If the watch spring pessary is used it is compressed into an elliptical shape and held in an introducer or by tying a piece of tape round it and clipping the tape with a pair of forceps. When the pessary has been introduced the forceps are released and the tape removed.

All patients who are wearing pessaries other than the perspex type should have a daily vaginal douche and may be taught to carry out this treatment themselves. Patients should also be given instructions as to when they should see their doctor for changing or removing the pessary. A rubber pessary may need changing every six weeks, a vulcanite pessary may be left for three months. Any patient who experiences pain or discomfort should be advised to report to her doctor as soon as possible.

25

Examination and Treatment of the Ear, Throat, Nose and Eye: Neurological Examination

Examination of the Ear

Requirements:

> Head mirror.
> Lamp.
> Aural specula of various sizes.
> Angular aural forceps.
> Small wool swabs.
> Receptacle for soiled swabs.

An electric auriscope may be used in place of the ordinary speculum, and the head mirror and lamp will not then be required.

The patient should sit sideways with the ear to be examined opposite the doctor. The light from the lamp is directed so that it shines on the head mirror.

If the auditory meatus is full of wax, the doctor will order the ear to be syringed before the examination can be completed.

To Syringe an Ear

Requirements:

> An aural syringe. A metal syringe may be used, or a Higginson's bulb syringe with a straight Eustachian catheter attached.
> Lotion (half-strength boracic acid lotion or sodium bicarbonate, 1 teaspoonful to water 1 pint).
> Lotion thermometer. The lotion should be prepared at 100° F. and injected at body temperature; if it is not the correct temperature the patient is likely to feel giddy and nauseated.

Angular aural forceps.
Wool swabs.
Mackintosh.
Towel.
Kidney-shaped receiver.
Receptacles for soiled swabs and instruments.
Head mirror and lamp.

The patient's clothes should be protected by the mackintosh and towel placed round his neck. He should sit upright if possible and hold the kidney dish under the ear.

The nurse should wear the head mirror and arrange the lamp so that it will shine on the mirror.

The syringe is filled with the lotion and air expelled.

The pinna of the ear should be pulled upwards and backwards to straighten the meatus and the flow of the lotion directed along the floor of the canal. When a piece of wax has been removed, the ear should be gently cleaned with a piece of wool on the angular forceps and the meatus examined to see if it is clear.

If the wax is hard, drops may be ordered to soften it; sodium bicarbonate or oil may be used.

After syringing a little ointment may be wiped round the meatus to prevent soreness.

A metal ear syringe should be handled with care. If dented, this will interfere with the smooth working of the plunger and there is danger that force may be used in pushing the plunger home, resulting in damage to the ear. The syringe should always be examined before use, to make sure that the plunger is working smoothly and evenly.

Examination of the Throat and Larynx
Requirements:

Head mirror.
Lamp.
Tongue depressor.
Tongue cloths or folded pieces of gauze or linen.
Laryngeal and post-nasal mirrors.
Spirit lamp and matches.
Local anæsthetic.
De Vilbiss spray.
Receptacles for used mirrors and instruments and for soiled swabs.

To Swab or Paint the Throat

Requirements:

> Tongue depressor.
> Cotton wool swabs on an applicator or held by forceps.
> A throat brush may be used in place of wool swabs.
> The throat paint and a small gallipot.
> Receptacles for used instruments and soiled swabs.

A good light is essential, and a hand lamp or a torch may be required.

The tongue depressor should be placed over the centre of the tongue, pushing it down gently into the floor of the mouth. It should not be placed too far back, as this is likely to make the patient retch.

The applications commonly ordered are glycerin and tannic acid, or Mandl's paint, a preparation of iodine, glycerin and peppermint.

Examination of the Nose and Nasopharynx

Requirements:

> Head mirror.
> Lamp.
> Nasal specula.
> Angular dressing forceps.
> Post-nasal mirrors.
> Tongue depressor.
> Spirit lamp and matches.
> Cotton wool.
> Cotton wool applicators or swab-holding forceps.
> Pieces of gauze.
> Receptacles for used mirrors and instruments and for soiled swabs.

For examinations of the throat, nose and nasopharynx when the patient is sitting up the nurse should steady the head with a hand on each side of the forehead, standing behind the patient so that he does not tend to back away from the examining surgeon.

Probes or wooden applicators dressed with special long-fibre cotton wool are frequently required in nose and throat work. These applicators can be bought ready for use or may be prepared by taking a small flat piece of wool, applying it to the edge of the applicator and twisting it tightly round, afterwards giving the wool a pull to make sure that it is firmly applied. Applicators should be dressed immediately before they are required, if prepared beforehand, they are liable to unwind.

Examination of the Eye. Examination of the interior of the eye with the ophthalmoscope is a procedure frequently carried out by the doctor in the general medical wards of a hospital, as well as by the ophthalmic surgeon in the eye department.

Requirements:

> An electrically illuminated ophthalmoscope is usually used.
>
> Small tray with eye drops and dropper.
>
> Small cotton wool swabs or folded lint squares.
>
> Receiver.

The following solutions may be ordered to dilate the pupil before the examination: homatropine 2 per cent., cocaine 4 per cent. or a mixture of 2 per cent. homatropine with 1 per cent. cocaine. No eye drops should be used without specific orders. The instillation of a mydriatic (a drug which dilates the pupil) into the eye of a patient suffering from glaucoma may cause blindness. Eserine drops may be ordered after the examination as a myotic to contract the pupil.

To Instil Drops into the Eye. The patient's head should be tilted well back and he should be directed to look up. One or two drops are then instilled into the lower part of the conjunctival sac, avoiding the cornea, which is the most sensitive part. The patient should be directed to close the eye for a few minutes. The lids should be gently wiped, taking the swab from the inner to the outer canthus. The dropper should never be allowed to touch the eye or the eyelashes.

To Irrigate the Eye

Requirements:

> A special glass irrigator known as an undine.
>
> Lotion at a temperature of 100° F. (Boracic lotion and normal saline solution are very commonly used; in cases of purulent conjunctivitis 1–8,000 perchloride of mercury may be ordered.)

Cotton wool or lint swabs.
Mackintosh cape.
Towel.
A receiver for the lotion.
A receptacle for used swabs.

Method. If the patient is in bed, all the pillows but one should be removed so that the patient lies flat with the head

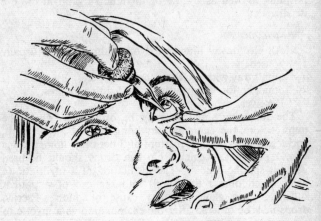

FIG. 56.—INSTILLATION OF DROPS.

tilted back. If he is sitting up in a chair, the head should be tilted back and inclined a little towards the affected side. The towel and mackintosh are arranged to protect the patient's clothing and the receiver arranged to catch the lotion. The patient may hold this himself.

The lotion from the irrigator may be allowed to flow over the cheek first, and is then directed in a steady stream from the inner towards the outer canthus of the eye, taking care that the undine does not touch the eye or the eyelashes. It should be held 1½ inches above the eye. The lids should be separated. If they are glued together with sticky discharge, this should be done very gently after well moistening the edges of the lids with lotion. The lids and the surrounding skin should be dried with swabs when the irrigation is completed. An antiseptic ointment for the lids, to be applied after the treatment, may be ordered, such as yellow oxide of mercury. This is applied to the edges of the lids by means of a glass rod.

In all cases where the eye is acutely red or there is any purulent discharge the nurse should observe the following precautions:

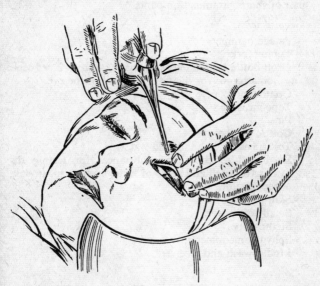

FIG. 57.—IRRIGATION OF UPPER CONJUNCTIVAL SAC WITH UPPER LID EVERTED.

(1) She should not directly touch with her fingers either the eye or any articles soiled with the discharge.

(2) If both eyes are to be treated, the cleaner eye should be attended to first.

(3) The nurse's hands must be very thoroughly washed after completing the treatment, the nurse being especially careful not to touch her own eye before doing this.

(4) The patient should be warned not to touch his eyes, and to keep all washing utensils, handkerchiefs and towels separate.

Neurological Examination

The examination of patients suffering from disease or

injury of the nervous system includes examination of the interior of the eye by means of an ophthalmoscope and testing of responses to sensory stimuli and reflex muscle responses.

The patient should undress for this examination and wear a pair of short "examination pants."

Requirements:

Patella hammer.

Tuning fork.

Drop bottle containing a mydriatic, such as 2 per cent. homatropine for dilating the pupil of the eye.

Ophthalmoscope.

Tape measure.

Pins.

Cotton wool mops.

Test tubes for hot and cold water.

Small bottles containing substances for testing the sense of smell and sense of taste, such as sugar, salt, peppermint.

Skin pencil.

Small soft brush.

Stethoscope.

Sphygmomanometer.

Mouth wash and receiver.

26

X-Ray Examinations: The use of Radioactive Substances in Diagnosis and Treatment

Preparation of the Patient for X-Ray Examination

THE wishes of the radiologist must be ascertained and carried out in all special examinations, and as several different methods are in use it is only possible to give some indication of the general lines of the preparation in each case.

The patient should be taken to the X-ray department suitably clad, so that the part to be examined can be readily bared of clothing without undue exposure of the patient. If the patient is allowed to keep on one garment during the examination of the chest or abdomen, this garment should be of cotton or flannel and the only fastenings should be tapes. Bone buttons and metal hooks will cast a shadow and linen buttons usually have a metal ring.

Any metal material or substance containing metal salts will obstruct the passage of X-rays and cast a shadow on the film, the only metal which will not materially interfere with the examination is aluminium.

Lead lotion, Elastoplast and kaolin are examples of materials which will obscure the X-ray picture of the underlying tissues. Wet plaster of Paris offers a greater obstruction than the same material when thoroughly dry, so that a plaster splint should, if possible be allowed to dry before the patient is X-rayed.

It is essential that the patient should remain quite still during the time of the exposure of the film, as any movement renders the radiograph hazy and valueless. The nurse should reassure a nervous patient and endeavour to make him understand that the examination is not in any way painful or harmful.

11+

Examination of the Renal Tract

The aim in the preparation for this examination is to have
the intestine emptied of both fæces and flatus, both of which
may render the examination useless by obscuring the kidney
shadow.

The patient is usually given an aperient such as Dulcolax
forty-eight or thirty-six hours before the examination, and
kept on a very light diet, or on a strict fluid diet. He is
allowed nothing after midnight on the morning of the
examination. Charcoal biscuits are sometimes given to
absorb the intestinal gas, and an injection of pituitrin may be
ordered half an hour before the examination. If the patient
is allowed to be out of bed and walking about, there is less
likelihood of an accumulation of gas in the intestine than if
he is completely confined to bed.

Pyelography

Retrograde Pyelography. A cystoscope is passed into
the bladder and a ureteric catheter opaque to X-rays passed
along the ureter into the pelvis of the kidney to be examined.
The injection of an opaque fluid into the pelvis of the kidney
is made through the ureteric catheter. A sterile solution of
sodium iodide 10 or 20 per cent. and a water soluble preparation of iodine, iodoxyl (proprietary name, Pyelectan Retrograde) are the two opaque media used for this purpose.
The radiographs are taken when the pelvis of the kidney is
filled with the solution.

Intravenous Pyelography (Excretion Pyelography). An
iodine compound, either diodone or iodoxyl is injected
intravenously: when excreted in the urine it is opaque to
X-rays, and will therefore cast a shadow of the renal pelves
when it fills these structures.

The tray for intravenous injection is taken to the X-ray
department with the patient, and the injection made while
the patient is on the examination table. Successive films
are taken from five minutes after the injection is completed.

Examination of the Lumbar Spine, Sacrum and Pelvis

The patient is usually prepared as for a renal tract
examination.

Examination of the Gall-Bladder

A radiograph of the gall-bladder may be taken after the same preparation of the patient as that necessary for X-ray of the urinary tract. In addition, however an examination is carried out after the patient has been given a dye which is excreted in the bile and renders it opaque. This procedure is known as cholecystography. The contrast medium generally used for oral administration is Telepaque, containing 66 per cent. iodine.

The routine followed may vary with the wishes of the radiologist, but the following is an outline of one method used extending over a period of three days.

On the first day a vegetable aperient is given, the dose will depend on the patient's habit with regard to laxatives but should be sufficient to ensure that the bowels act. On the second day the patient takes a low-residue diet excluding green vegetables, cereals and whole meal bread. After supper the dose of Telepaque is given and no food or drink is allowed until the X-ray film has been taken on the following morning.

The patient attends the X-ray Department at the stated time. He may be required to return after one or two hours for further films. When the gall-bladder, filled with dye containing bile, is demonstrated radiographically, the patient is given a meal with a high fat content, *e.g.* an egg, milk with added cream and a liberal amount of butter on toast or bread. One hour later he attends the department for the final examination.

Intravenous Cholecystogram. When the oral method fails to outline the gall-bladder a cholecystangiography may be performed. This is an examination of the gall-bladder and bile ducts by an intravenous opaque injection (Biligrafin) which contains a higher percentage of iodine than the oral preparation, and results in a higher concentration in the biliary and commen bile ducts.

Cholangiography. The bile ducts can be demonstrated by the same intravenous method in patients who have had the gall-bladder removed.

Preparation for Intravenous Cholecystangiography and Cholangiography

1st day. An aperient (vegetable laxative) is given the patient two nights before the X-ray examination.

2nd day. A low residue diet is taken by the patient. No green vegetables, cereals or wholemeal bread. Nothing to eat or drink after midnight.

3rd day. A preliminary film is taken and is examined. If this is satisfactory, *i.e.* if the preparation is adequate and the gall-bladder area is clear of intestinal contents, the intravenous injection is given. The first film is taken 15 minutes later, and films are then taken at varying intervals depending on the rate of concentration of the opaque medium in the gall-bladder. When the concentration is adequate, a fatty meal is given and a further film is taken.

For a cholangiogram films are taken in the same manner up to about 45 minutes after the injection. No fatty meal is given as there is no gall-bladder present.

Opaque Meal Examination of the Alimentary Tract

The substance used to render the alimentary tract opaque to X-rays is barium sulphate. It is insoluble in water, and therefore is commonly prepared in the form of a suspension containing 4 oz. of barium sulphate in 20 oz. of the preparation.

No aperient should be given within 24 hours of the examination, and any medicine containing bismuth should be discontinued for three days beforehand.

No food or drink should be taken within six hours of the examination. If the examination is for the stomach and duodenum only it may be completed in three hours. If the entire alimentary tract is to be examined, the procedure will extend over 24 or 48 hours, in some cases longer.

As a general rule no food is allowed until the stomach is seen to be empty, and no aperients or other medicines or enemas are allowed until the examination is completed.

An opaque meal examination may be required for an infant, usually in the investigation of pyloric stenosis. In place of the barium preparation 1 oz. of bismuth powder is added to the infant's feed and given at the normal feeding time. No preparation is required.

Examination of the Appendix

An aperient is given 36 hours before the examination and no food or fluid is allowed within 6 hours of the barium meal. The first radiograph is taken 6 hours after the patient

has taken the barium mixture and again no food or drink
is allowed during this period. Some radiologists order
120 gr. of magnesium sulphate to be given 2 hours after the
barium meal. After the first radiographs the patient may
have his normal diet but no aperient may be given until the
examination is completed, which is usually at the end of
24 hours.

Opaque Enema Examination of the Colon

An aperient is given 36 hours before and a colon wash-
out 4 hours before the examination.

The barium mixture for the opaque enema can be conveniently prepared by adding an equal quantity of warm
water to the suspension used for the barium meal examination. At least 3 pints will be required.

The enema is allowed to run in slowly through a rectal
tube while the radiologist examines the patient under the
fluoroscopic screen. The mixture must be at body temperature and should be continually stirred during the administration.

The patient may be required in the X-ray department
24 hours after the enema has been given, and in this case no
aperient or enema must be given without special instruction.

The patient is usually allowed a cup of tea on the morning
of the examination and his usual diet afterwards.

Bronchography

This examination is carried out after an opaque medium
has been injected into the bronchus. The object is to
obtain a picture of the bronchi and their branches and
is a useful diagnostic aid in suspected carcinoma of the
bronchus and in the condition of bronchiectasis. Opaque
media used are either iodine in poppyseed oil (Lipiodol and
Neo-Hydriol) or Dionosil in water or oil.

The injection may be done by puncturing the cricothyroid membrane and so entering the trachea, by dropping
the oil into the trachea from the mouth with a special
syringe and curved catheter or by means of a catheter
through the nose or mouth.

Requirements. (1) *For injection by the cricothyroid route.*

A 2-ml. record syringe and hypodermic needles.

Bronchography syringe and special needle (Fig. 58).

Local anæsthetic.
Lipiodol or Dionosil.
Sterile towels, swabs and small gauze dressing.
Spirit or cetrimide for cleaning the skin.
Mackintosh.
Bowl for soiled swabs.
Sand bag.

The patient may lie on his back with no pillow under the head and the sand bag under the shoulders, or be sitting up with the head extended.

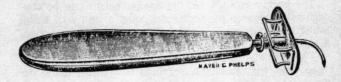

FIG. 58.—FIELD'S BRONCHOGRAPHY NEEDLE.
(Child's size)

(2) *For the oral method:*

Bronchography syringe with curved dropper.
Pieces of folded gauze or tongue cloths.
Tongue depressor.
De Vilbiss spray.
Local anæsthetic.
Mackintosh.
Towel.
Vomit bowl.
Lipiodol standing in a bowl of water.

(3) *For the catheter method.* In addition to the above requirements:

Laryngeal mirror.
Head mirror.
Spirit lamp.
5-ml. syringe.
Acorn attachment to fit the syringe to the catheters.
Two elastic gum catheters, size 6 and 7, English gauge, sterile.
Curved applicator with wool for anæsthetizing the larynx.

Preparation of the Patient and Special Precautions. The patient is allowed no food within six hours of the examination if the opaque medium is administered by the oral or intratracheal catheter methods on account of the tendency to vomit.

A sedative such as codeine and a hypodermic injection of atropine may be ordered half an hour before the examination.

The patient, with his head supported, should sit on a low chair facing the operator.

After the injection the patient must be warned not to cough until the X-ray films have been taken.

The patient is not allowed any food or fluid until the effects of the local anæsthetic have completely disappeared and the cough reflex is re-established. If the patient tries to swallow while the larynx is still anæsthetized the food or fluid may pass down the trachea into the lungs.

Salpingography

This is an X-ray examination of the Fallopian tube after the injection of iodized oil or diodone viscous solution (Viskiosol Six) into the cavity of the uterus. The object of the examination is to demonstrate the patency of the Fallopian tubes, stenosis or closure of the tubes being one of the causes of sterility in women.

The injection of the oil is made on the X-ray table and the patient is usually placed in the lithotomy position. The examination does not as a rule entail any preparation other than the administration of an aperient 36 hours previously if necessary. The patient should empty the bladder immediately before the injection is made.

Requirements:

Container of iodized oil standing in a bowl of hot water
Sterile instruments, vaginal speculum, vaginal retractor, two pairs of sponge-holding forceps, two pairs of vulsellum forceps, intra-uterine nozzle (*e.g.* Fosdike's) to fit the special oil syringe.
Sterile swabs, towels and vulval pad.
Sterile gloves and gown for the doctor.
Bowl of lotion, *e.g.* Bradosol 1 in 2000 solution.
Mackintosh.
Receptacles for soiled dressings and instruments.

Radiographs are taken at the completion of the injection and at the end of 24 hours. During this period the patient should not be given an aperient or an enema.

Ventriculography

This examination is carried out after the injection of air into the lateral ventricles of the brain.

The injection of air is carried out by the surgeon in the theatre, and the patient is afterwards transferred to the X-ray department for the radiographs.

The preparation of the patient is the same as for trephining the skull; the scalp must be shaved and the skin prepared.

Encephalography

This is another method of investigating the position and shape of the ventricles. With the patient sitting astride a chair a lumbar puncture is performed. Cerebrospinal fluid is withdrawn and 5 ml. of air is injected. The air rises, as it is lighter than the fluid in the subarachnoid space, and fills the ventricles. The radiographs are then taken.

Examination of the Cardiovascular System

Angiocardiography. This procedure is an investigation of the heart and great blood-vessels. An intravenous injection of 30 to 50 ml. of an opaque iodine-containing compound (Diodone) is made into a vein at the elbow. The fluid is injected as quickly as possible and a series of films is taken rapidly to show the passage of the opaque medium through the heart and the great blood-vessels attached to it.

Another method used is the introduction of a catheter into a vein or artery through which the iodine compound is injected. For investigation of the aorta in cases of suspected coarctation the catheter is introduced into the right brachial or into the common carotid artery. For examination of the right side of the heart in cases of Fallot's tetralogy or of patent ductus arteriosus the catheter is introduced into the right cephalic vein at the elbow or into the saphenous vein of the thigh.

Catheterization of the Heart. This procedure is carried out by introducing a long opaque catheter into a vein in the right elbow and watching its passage under the fluorescent screen through the innominate vein, the superior vena cava, the right auricle and the right ventricle to the pulmonary artery. Samples of blood for examination of the oxygen content are withdrawn from the chambers of the heart.

For these investigations a local anæsthetic is used for adults, but a general anæsthetic may be required for a child.

Tests for sensitivity to cocaine and iodine may be carried out beforehand.

Therapeutic Use of X-rays

The term "deep X-ray treatment" implies the use of penetrating X-rays produced by the bombardment of a target by electrons travelling at high speed. The source of the energy required for this is high-voltage electricity, of the order of 180 to 100,000 kilovolts. This form of treatment is most frequently used in cases of malignant growth and many of the patients are treated by this method.

Many require a large dose spread over a period of several weeks in order that a lethal dose can be delivered at the site of the growth without producing either generalized ill-effects or localized damage to the skin and surrounding tissues.

However carefully the scheme of treatment is devised the tissues surrounding the growth are likely to suffer at least some temporary ill-effects and this is especially true of the skin. Therefore great care is required during and for some weeks after the treatment. The skin of the areas treated must not be subjected to any chemical or physical irritants, therefore washing with soap and water, antiseptic lotions and hot or cold applications must be avoided. If a male patient is receiving treatment to the face or neck, shaving is usually forbidden for a time and the friction of a closely fitting stiff collar should be avoided. Mucous membrane reacts to radiation in much the same way as skin and some temporary damage to mucus-secreting cells will occur. If the mouth is included in the treatment area there will be a diminution in the secretion of both saliva and mucus. The patient may be very disinclined to eat on account of the discomfort and pain caused by a dry mouth and must be helped and encouraged as much as possible. Frequent non-irritating fluids to drink and frequent mouth washes will help. If the mouth is painful, lozenges containing a local anæsthetic—e.g. benzocaine—may be ordered, or aspirin gargles may give relief.

11*

General effects of radiation are not usually marked when divided dosage is used spread over a period of weeks, but were fairly common in the early days of X-ray treatment when a single large dose was used. However, some patients may complain of loss of appetite, nausea, inability to sleep and general depression.

Radium Therapy

Radium is a naturally occurring element which spontaneously emits radiations of short wave-length. Radium is chiefly used in the form of its salt, radium sulphate, and in the form of the emanation or gas (radon) which is given off from it. The salt is placed in needles or sometimes in larger containers and the emanation is collected in radon "seeds."

Methods of Application

Surface Application. The needles or applicators are embedded in a suitable mould made of Columba paste or Stent's dental composition, or may be attached to sorbo rubber or other suitable material which can be accurately applied to the desired area.

Interstitial Irradiation. Needles or radon seeds are inserted into the tissues.

Cavitary Irradiation. Applicators are placed inside natural cavities of the body—*e.g.* the vagina and cervical canal.

Rules and Precautions to be Observed in the Handling of Radium

Radium needles or containers, including radon seeds, should never be touched by hand but must always be manipulated with long-handled forceps the handles of which are covered with rubber. When radium is removed from the safe and carried to and from the theatre a lead-lined box with a long carrying handle should be used for its transport.

The threading of needles and the preparation of applicators must be carried out on a special table provided with a lead screen. Proximity to the radium must be for as short a time as possible.

The time at which the radium treatment is begun and the time at which it is due to be terminated must be carefully noted. The success of the treatment and the safety of the patient depend on careful calculation of the dosage to be employed. The time during which the radium is in contact with the tissues is one factor in these calculations.

Careful checking of the radium is essential. The amount of radium, the number and size of the needles used are entered on a record card; unused containers are checked and returned to the radium safe.

Radioactive Isotopes

Isotopes are variations of an element which have identical chemical properties but different atomic weights. Most elements have at least two isotopes. The radioactive isotopes of certain elements which are now being used in medical treatment are artificially produced by the bombardment of the nuclei of the atoms in an atomic pile. The radioactive isotopes used in medicine are in fact by-products of the atomic research stations.

Examples of the medical use of radioactive isotopes:

Radioactive iodine in the treatment of carcinoma of the thyroid gland. The radioactive iodine is given by mouth and absorbed into the blood stream from the alimentary tract. From the blood it is deposited in the thyroid gland and there acts as a source of localized radiation.

Radioactive phosphorus. This substance has been found to be effective in the treatment of polycythæmia, a condition in which the blood contains an excessive number of red cells. The phosphorus may be given by mouth or by intravenous injection.

Radioactive cobalt. This has a long "life" compared with most other radioactive isotopes. It is now being used in place of radium or as an alternative to deep X-ray in a "bomb" or beam unit in the treatment of malignant disease.

Radioactive gold. This isotope is used locally in the peritoneal or pleural cavities in cases of malignant disease where secondary deposits cause large peritoneal or pleural effusions necessitating frequent aspiration.

Radioactive Tracers

Radioactive isotopes are useful assistants in solving physiological and medical problems. Very minute quantities can be traced in the body by means of a delicate instrument, the Geiger counter. For example, radioactive iodine is used to assess the activity of the thyroid gland. A small dose is given by mouth and the Geiger counter is set up in position over the thyroid area and will record the arrival of the radioactive isotope in the tissues of the gland. If there is no active thyroid tissue no iodine will be taken up; if there is enlargement and/or increased activity of the gland the absorption of the iodine will be more rapid than normal.

Precautions

All persons working with radioactive substances or X-rays must observe the regulations laid down for their protection or their health will sooner or later be affected. Prolonged exposure to even small doses of radiation will damage the bone marrow and eventually diminish the supply of blood cells. The germ plasm of the ovaries and testes is damaged by radiation and sterility may result. In the early days of the use of X-rays repeated exposure of the hands caused destruction of the skin, ulceration and later malignant changes.

In the handling of radioactive isotopes similar precautions are required as in dealing with other forms of radiation, but in addition there is the danger of contamination with radioactive particles.

When patients are receiving doses of radioactive iodine some of the material will be excreted in the urine. Nursing staff dealing with bedpans and urinals should wear protective clothing and rubber gloves. Should there be any suspicion of contamination of the hands or any skin area a thorough washing with soap and water must be immediately carried out. The radioactive urine must not be emptied directly into the sewerage system. The radioactivity rapidly decays, however (the exact period of time which must elapse before the isotope is inactive varies with the different elements), and after storage for the appropriate length of time the urine can be discarded. Urine awaiting disposal can be stored in suitable large bottles or tanks in lead-lined cupboards.

The following regulations are an example of the precautions which the nursing staff must observe in caring for a patient who is receiving treatment of the thyroid gland with radioactive iodine.

China. Separate china and cutlery will be used for all

patients having had radioactive iodine. The china is green-bordered. All cutlery and glassware is marked with green paint. It may be washed in the kitchen, but in different water from other china. A separate dish mop and towel will be used and all cutlery is to be soaked in half strength 1 per cent. potassium iodide for $\frac{1}{4}$ hour before being washed.

Mouthwash utensils. All utensils are marked with green paint.

Urine. Each patient has his own marked bedpan.
Urine is placed by patients in, and saved in, 24 hourly bottles behind lead shielding until it is safe for disposal. These urine bottles are then dealt with by the laboratory staff.

Fæces. No precautions are required.

Vomit and sputum. Any material vomited or expectorated within the first 48 hours of a dose is saved in a lead-lined cupboard.

Contaminated bedding, etc. This is saved for monitoring, any urine spills being notified.

Hands. In order to avoid contamination of the hands rubber gloves are worn when attending to patients who are receiving therapy doses. The gloves must be worn for bed-making and for giving attention to the patient during the first 3 days after a therapeutic dose and during the first 7 days when dealing with the patient's urine. Gloves should be washed on the hands before they are removed. The hands must be washed after removing the gloves and again before eating or smoking.

Nurses should avoid exposing their hands for longer than a minute or two to the radiation from the neck region.

27

Special Procedures and Examination

Exploration of the Chest for Fluid in the Pleural Cavity

Exploration and, where necessary, aspiration of the pleural cavity are used in diagnosis and the treatment of a pleural effusion. Such an effusion may be an inflammatory exudate as in pleurisy accompanying pneumonia, or a transudate such as the fluid which collects as part of a generalized œdema in congestive heart failure.

Requirements:

Local anæsthetic.
2-ml. record syringe and needles.
Exploring syringe and long needles.
Instrument forceps.
Sterile swabs and towels.
Cetrimide, ether or spirit.
Gauze dressing.
Collodion.
Mackintosh.
Sterile test tubes (for the fluid withdrawn).
Receptacle for dirty dressings.
Hypodermic tray with stimulants.

Position of the Patient. He may lean forward, resting on a bed table, or lie with the affected side uppermost and several pillows placed to support the shoulder on which he is lying.

Aspirating the Chest (i.e. Removing a Collection of Fluid from the Pleural Cavity)

Aspiration Using a Two-way Syringe (Fig. 59). The general requirements are as enumerated above with the addition of a two-way syringe with connections and two sterile measure jugs.

Martin's syringe (Fig. 59) is one type of two-way syringe used for aspiration of the chest. This syringe has a bayonet fitting and is supplied with a trocar and cannula and a sharp needle. A piece of rubber tubing is attached to one arm of the nozzle through which the fluid drawn up into the syringe is ejected into the measure jug.

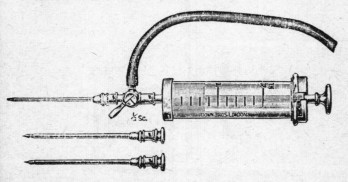

FIG. 59.—MARTIN'S SYRINGE.

Artificial Pneumothorax and Pneumoperitoneum

The introduction of air into the pleural space or into the peritoneal cavity may be undertaken in order to produce collapse of a lung, or part of a lung, in the treatment of tuberculosis. Air replacement may be required following the withdrawal of fluid in case of pleural effusion.

Requirements:

Local anæsthetic.
Hypodermic syringe and needles.
Cetrimide, surgical spirit or ether.
Sterile towels, swabs and gauze.
Sterile forceps and scissors.
Collodion or mastic for sealing the gauze dressing.
Hypodermic tray, stimulants and adrenaline.
Cheatle's instrument forceps.
Receptacle for soiled swabs.
Artificial pneumothorax apparatus and primary trocar
    and cannula or "refill" needle as required.

There are several varieties of artificial pneumothorax apparatus in use. One of the simplest and most convenient is Stott's apparatus which is shown in Fig. 60. Two glass cylinders (A) are fixed to two horizontal bars both of which

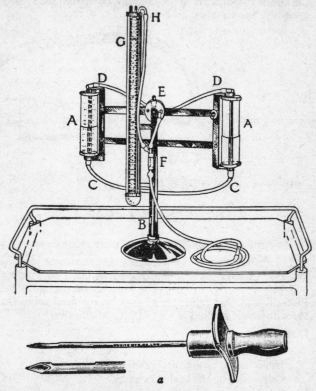

FIG. 60.—STOTT'S ARTIFICIAL PNEUMOTHORAX APPARATUS
a. Morland's refill needle (full size).

are pivoted on a central column (B) thus permitting a "see-saw" movement of the cylinders. A piece of rubber tubing (C) joins the two cylinders at their bases. Two rubber tubes (D) connect the cylinders with the inlet and outlet ports respectively at the slide valve (E). Air entering passes through a small filter at the inlet; air passing out goes through the main filter (F). The exit of this filter has two connections; one via the U-tube (H) to the manometer (G), the other connection via tubing to the induction cannula or refill needle, whichever is being used.

When the apparatus is assembled the graduated glass cylinder is filled with water to the 200-ml. mark. Usually an antiseptic is added (*e.g.* a 1–40 solution of phenol is used in place of plain water). The U-tube is filled with water which may be coloured with an aniline dye. The tubing connecting the slide valve and the main filter must be attached to the positive part (marked "+" on the apparatus). The cylinders, valve filters and tubing can be dismantled for cleaning and sterilization by boiling. A small handle at the right-hand end of the upper horizontal bar can also be removed and sterilized; this handle enables the operator to alter the position of the cylinders during the procedure.

For the primary induction a cannula fitted with two stilettes is used. One stilette has a sharp end and is used to penetrate the chest wall down to the pleura; it is then changed for the blunt stilette to penetrate the pleura. For a refill a hollow bevelled needle, *e.g.* Morland refill needle, is used (Fig. 60A).

Preparation of the Patient for a Primary Artificial Pneumothorax. Morphine or codeine is usually ordered to be given half an hour previously. The patient should lie on the sound side, with the arm on the affected side above his head and with the head lower than the chest; a firm pillow is placed under the chest and no pillow is allowed at the head.

The skin over the site of the injection is cleaned and painted with iodine, and the local anæsthetic is injected. After the trocar is withdrawn the skin puncture is sealed with a gauze and collodion dressing.

Refill. A local anæsthetic may be used. The patient is not usually given a narcotic. After the needle is withdrawn the puncture is sealed with a gauze and collodion dressing.

Since the introduction of chemotherapeutic drugs successful in the treatment of tuberculosis, the induction of a pneumothorax in the treatment of pulmonary tuberculosis is now comparatively infrequent.

Tapping the Abdomen (Paracentesis Abdominis).

Tapping may be needed in order to withdraw fluid from the

peritoneal cavity (ascites) in cases of cardiac or liver diseases and in malignant conditions.

   Requirements:

   Local anæsthetic.
   Record syringe and needles.
   Cetrimide, ether or spirit.
   Sterile swabs and towels.
   Gauze and wool dressings.
   Many-tailed bandage or abdominal binder.
   Adhesive plaster.
   Pail or other receptacle to stand at the side of the bed
      for the fluid.
   Mackintosh.
   Receptacles for used swabs and instruments.
   Instrument forceps.
   A small scalpel or tenotomy knife.
   Hypodermic tray with stimulants.

Tapping Apparatus.

   (1) Ascites trocar and cannula, with a long piece of rubber tubing attached to the side outlet.

   (2) Southey's tubing and fine trocar and cannula.

   When the Southey's tube is used the trocar should have the small shield screwed into place and the tubing should be attached to the end of the cannula. The trocar should be pushed through the rubber tubing (holding this stretched) so that its end protrudes just below the end of the cannula.

   It is important that the fine tubing should be new and in good condition; if at all perished it will lose its elasticity, and therefore the small hole made by the trocar will not close up when the trocar is removed.

   Preparation of the Patient. Immediately before the tapping the bladder must be emptied and a catheterization may be needed.

   The patient should sit upright supported with pillows. The bandage or binder should be placed in position so that it can be applied as soon as the trocar and cannula are inserted. If a large trocar and cannula are used, the fluid drains quickly and the nurse should tighten the binder frequently. If a Southey's tube is used the fluid drains much more slowly. Two small pieces of adhesive strapping will be required to keep the small shield in position.

Tapping the Legs

The commoner causes of gross œdema of the legs are cardiac failure and nephritis.

Requirements:

A small scalpel.
Southey's small trocars and cannulæ (two for each leg are usually required).
Capillary rubber drainage tubing.
Skin preparation tray.
Local anæsthetic.
Record syringe and needles.
Sterile lint, towels and dressings.
Dissecting forceps.
Scissors.
Instrument forceps in jar.
Porringers or small jars for receiving the fluid.
Receptacles for soiled swabs and instruments.
Mackintoshes.

Preparation of the Apparatus. The tubing is fitted on to the cannulæ as for paracentesis abdominis with Southey's tubes, but the small metal shields are omitted.

A few ounces of 5 per cent. phenol or similar disinfectant are placed in the jars for receiving the fluid.

Preparation of the Patient. As a general rule an endeavour is made to drain fluid from other parts of the body into the legs prior to the tapping. To achieve this the patient's legs should hang down below the level of the trunk for two or three days beforehand.

The skin on the outer aspect of the legs is prepared.

A local anæsthetic may be injected into the skin surrounding the site for the insertion of the cannulæ.

When the tubes have been inserted, small pieces of lint are slipped under the ends of the cannulae to prevent pressure on the skin. The tubes are kept in place by small pieces of adhesive strapping and covered by sterile dressings. The ends of the rubber drainage tubes are placed in the jars.

The tubes may be left in twenty-four hours or longer; during this time the dressings should be changed twice a day, or more often if necessary. After the tubes have been removed the punctures must be covered with sterile dressings until they are healed.

As an alternative method, small scarifications may be made in the œdematous tissue.

Lumbar Puncture

Lumbar puncture is carried out in order to obtain samples of cerebro-spinal fluid and to measure the pressure of the fluid. The procedure is also used when drugs are given by intrethecal injection.

Requirements:

> Lumbar puncture needles. If the pressure of the cerebrospinal fluid is to be measured, a needle with a tap and side piece is used. A small piece of rubber tubing to fit the side piece and the glass manometer will be required. This tubing and the manometer must be sterilized.
>
> Sterile test tubes.
> Sterile swabs and towels.
> Local anæsthetic.
> Hypodermic syringe and needles.
> A small gauze dressing.
> Collodion.
> Dissecting forceps.
> Scissors.
> Instrument forceps in jar.
> Cetrimide, ether or spirit.
> Mackintosh.
> Receptacles for soiled swabs and instruments.

If drugs are to be injected a large record syringe and an adaptor to fit the lumbar puncture needle will be required.

A general anæsthetic may be required if the patient is restless or likely to have fits.

Position of the Patient. Usually the procedure is carried out with the patient lying on his side near the edge of the bed. The spine and the legs are flexed as far as possible in order to separate the intervertebral spaces. The usual site for the puncture is between the third and fourth lumbar vertebræ. It some cases the patient may be sitting up with the knees and spine flexed.

After the procedure the patient should be kept quiet and lying flat for several hours, as severe headache is likely to occur. This may be treated by raising the foot of the bed.

When specimens of the cerebrospinal fluid are collected for

pathological examination, the test tubes in which the fluid is collected should be immediately stoppered with sterile wool and taken to the laboratory. Care must be taken to see that the tubes are kept upright and the fluid not allowed to come in contact with the wool plugs.

Cisternal Puncture

The requirements are the same as for lumbar puncture, except that a special needle with the shaft marked in centimetres may be used.

The site for this puncture is the junction of the skull with the spin, and the skin over the area will usually require shaving.

Venesection

This procedure is dealt with under Blood Transfusion p. 234.

Bone Marrow Biopsy

In the investigation of some diseases of the blood a specimen of the red bone marrow is required and this is obtained either from the sternum or the iliac crest.

Requirements:

Ether, spirit or cetrimide for cleaning the skin.
Sterile swabs, towels and dressing.
Adhesive strapping or collodion.
Hypodermic syringe and needle for local anæsthetic.
2 per cent. Novocain or other local anæsthetic.
1-ml. syringe.
Sternal puncture needle with stilette. This is a hollow needle with a short bevelled point and an adjustable "stop" or guard.
Sterile test tube or small specimen bottle.

The patient is usually given a sedative, *e.g.* Seconal 200 mg. or Physeptone 10 mg. three-quarters to one hour before the procedure is carried out.

The patient should lie flat with the head extended and a small pillow under the shoulders.

A **Splenic Aspiration** is sometimes performed in cases of unexplained splenomegaly and in some blood diseases. For this a fine-gauge Harris's lumbar puncture needle may be used ,and a syringe for aspirating the specimen.

Liver Biopsy

Biopsy may be required in the investigation of liver disorders where physical and laboratory examinations have failed to give a diagnosis.

Requirements:

Alcohol, cetrimide or ether for cleaning the skin.

Sterile swabs and dressings.

Hypodermic syringe and needles for local anæsthetic, including a fine needle 3 inches in length.

Local anæsthetic, *e.g.* 2 per cent. solution of procaine.

Sterile scalpel.

Forceps.

Sterile gloves.

Liver biopsy needle, *e.g.* Silverman's or a modification of this type (see Fig. 61).

Collodion.

A small bottle containing formalin for the specimen.

Pathological examination request forms.

Receptacle for soiled swabs.

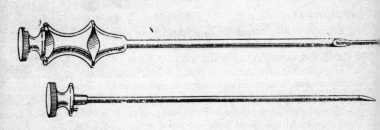

Fig. 61. Silverman's Liver Biopsy, Adult Size.

Preparation. The patient's blood group is ascertained and his blood is cross-matched. The hæmoglobin content, bleeding and clotting times and the prothrombin content of the blood are estimated. The examination is not usually carried out if the prothrombin content is below 70 per cent. of the normal.

Procedure. The patient lies on his back well over to the right side of the bed, the trunk is then slightly tilted to the right by placing a pillow under his left side.

Following the biopsy it is important to keep a close watch on the patient's condition as hæmorrhage may occur. A pulse chart should be kept for at least twelve hours.

Renal Biopsy

Renal biopsy may be useful in elucidating some cases of renal disease when other methods have failed to give a definite diagnosis.

Preparation of the Patient. An X-ray examination is carried out in order to determine the size of the kidneys. The patient's blood group is identified and his blood is cross-matched in case a transfusion is needed. The hæmoglobin is also estimated.

Procedure. The site of the biopsy is usually the lower pole of the right kidney. The patient lies in the prone position with a sandbag under the abdomen, this fixes the kidney against the dorsal surface of the body and helps to reduce the risk of hæmorrhage.

The position of the kidney is determined after the injection of a local anæsthetic, by a fine exploring needle.

The biopsy specimen is obtained by using a modified type of the Silverman's liver biopsy needle.

After renal biopsy has been performed it is important to keep a close watch for bleeding; a certain amount of hæmaturia is common, but even if slight it should be reported immediately.

28

Methods of Treatment: Local applications

Inhalations

Steam Kettle. The kettle is used in conjunction with a tent bed in the treatment of bronchitis. In a small room a screen round the head of the bed with a sheet over the top may replace the full tent.

An electric kettle is generally used, as there is a risk of fire if a spirit stove is used for heating.

The kettle should stand on a stool and the spout should be introduced either at the side or the foot of the tent.

The kettle should be filled with boiling water, and if a drug is ordered this is added to the water in the prescribed quantity. Compound tincture of benzoin is commonly used. The kettle usually requires filling every two hours, and should be refilled with boiling water. The air temperature in the tent should be 70° F.

If the patient is a child it is necessary to have some form of restraint, so that the child cannot get at any part of the kettle or come into close contact with the steam, or else the kettle should be sufficiently far from the cot to prevent this occurring.

Nelson's Inhaler. The earthenware inhaler should be half filled with boiling water to which the prescribed amount of menthol or tincture of benzoin is added. This is usually 60 minims of tincture of benzoin or a few crystals of menthol to 1 pint of water.

A flannel cover should be placed round the inhaler and the patient's shoulders should be covered with a shawl or small blanket. The patient is directed to put his lips to the mouth-piece and breathe in through the mouth and out through the nose.

A very satisfactory inhaler can be made by using a quart jug with a small towel twisted round the rim. The patient is directed to rest his mouth on the towel and breathe in the steam.

The treatment is chiefly ordered for inflammation of the upper air passages. Some authorities recommend that the hot water in the inhaler should not be hotter than 180° F A steam inhalation is not suitable for a patient who for any reason is unable to co-operate in the treatment.

Hot Applications

The effects of external application of heat are:

(1) Increase of the local blood supply in the superficial tissues.

(2) Increased number and activity of leucocytes in the part, favouring the removal of waste material and inflammatory exudate.

(3) Relaxation of the muscles.

Heat is very commonly employed to relieve pain and congestion.

A counter-irritant also produces a hyperæmia locally, usually these substances redden the skin more quickly than simple applications of heat. They also cause dilatation of the lymph vessels, and if sufficiently irritating will produce blistering.

Applications for the relief of pain are often combinations of heat and some irritant substance, so that hot applications and counter-irritants may be considered together.

Simple applications of heat which may succeed in relieving pain are hot-water bottles, a hot bath, bathing the part with hot water, or the use of an electric pad or radiant heat cradle.

When heat is used for the relief of severe pain, special care must be taken to guard against burning, as the patient who is suffering acutely will not feel the lesser discomfort of heat.

If a rubber hot-water bottle is used it should be very well protected with a thick cover and filled with water which will give the bottle a comfortable temperature. Boiling water should not be used.

Fomentation and Stupes

A fomentation is a simple method of applying heat locally but does not retain the heat for any length of time.

Requirements:

A piece of flannel of double or treble thickness.

A piece of protective material, such as jaconet, $\frac{1}{2}$ inch larger all round than the flannel.

A piece of gamgee or cotton wool $\frac{1}{2}$ inch larger than the jaconet. If jaconet is not obtainable, brown wool should be used instead of absorbent white wool.

A wringer made of strong cotton or linen material. In the home a strong kitchen towel makes a good wringer

A bowl.

A kettle of boiling water.

A flannel bandage or binder should be used to keep the application in position.

Place the flannel in the centre of the wringer and take care that the ends of the wringer lie outside the bowl, pour the boiling water over the flannel and wringer and then wring the flannel as dry as possible. Give it a quick shake to allow the steam to escape before applying.

The flannel is then covered with the jaconet and wool and bandaged in position.

The frequency with which the fomentation is changed will depend upon its size and thickness and the condition for which it is ordered. In some cases it will require changing every half-hour, in others every two hours will be sufficient.

When a fomentation is to be changed, the fresh application should be prepared and the old one removed (leaving the part covered with the piece of wool) before wringing out the fresh fomentation.

The effect of the hot moist application in relieving pain may be increased by the addition of a counter-irritant such as turpentine, or the addition of a drug which will act as a local analgesic, as, for example, opium or belladonna although the efficacy of these as local applications is open to question.

Turpentine Stupe.

Requirements. As for the medical fomentation, with the addition of the required amount of oil of turpentine, usually 1 to 4 drachms.

In order to prevent burning the turpentine must be distributed as evenly as possible, and for this reason it is sprinkled on the flannel before the boiling water is poured on.

Another method is to place the turpentine in a warm jug,

to pour on it 1 pint of boiling water, and then pour the mixture of water and turpentine over the flannel. The skin should be inspected, and when reddened the turpentine stupe should be removed and replaced by a simple fomentation or by a piece of warm cotton wool. As an average, thirty minutes will be as long as the stupe should be allowed to remain on the skin.

This treatment may be ordered for the relief of distension as well as the relief of pain.

Kaolin Poultice (Cataplasma Kaolini). The basis of this application is china clay, which contains, in addition, glycerin, menthol and methyl salicylate. It has analgesic as well as heat-retaining properties.

The kaolin poultice may be left on six to twelve hours, and this is a great advantage in cases where frequent applications are exhausting to the patient, and it has also the advantage of being light in weight.

Requirements:

Tin containing cataplasma kaolini.
Saucepan containing boiling water.
Lint or old linen (prepared as for a linseed poultice).
Palette knife.
Jug containing boiling water.
Poultice board.
Warmed plates, trays or dishes to carry the poultice to the bedside.

Place the tin containing the application in the saucepan and allow it to heat by keeping the water simmering for about twenty minutes. The contents of the tin should be stirred occasionally, so that the material is evenly heated all through.

Spread the poultice smoothly on the lint or linen, place it on a warm tray or plate, covered (do not roll or fold the poultice), and take it to the bedside. The heat of the application should be tested on the back of the hand before applying. Clay holds the heat for a long time, and unless the poultice is tested to make sure that it is not too hot there is a danger of burning the patient.

Leeches

Leeches are sometimes ordered for the relief of pain in acute eye conditions such as glaucoma and iritis. They are occasionally used in the treatment of pericarditis, and may be applied over the liver in congestive heart failure. They may also be used to assist the absorption of a hæmatoma.

Each leech will suck from 1 to 2 drachms of blood.

Leech bites may continue to bleed for some time after the leech has dropped off on account of the anticoagulant, hirudin, manufactured by the leech. A patient should not be left during the application, and every care should be taken to prevent the patient from seeing or feeling the leeches on the skin.

Requirements:

The required number of leeches.

A bowl with a cover.

Two or three test tubes two-thirds filled with cotton wool.

A piece of non-scented soap, some warm water in a bowl, and a few swabs.

A bowl containing 1-20 phenol lotion.

A bowl containing salt.

A piece of lint or oiled silk with a number of small hole cut in it corresponding to the number of leeches to be used.

Circular dressings of wool and gauze to apply to the bites.

Adhesive plaster.

Bandages.

A sheet of firm but thin paper.

A gallipot containing a small quantity of sweetened milk.

The skin is prepared by washing with soap and water. The piece of oiled silk is placed over the part to which the leeches are to be applied.

Leeches become disinclined to suck if they are handled or manipulated when being applied and a satisfactory method of avoiding this is to place them in a small pot containing water and covered by a lid in which holes have been made. When the test tube is held against the hole in the lid the leech will explore its way through the hole and into the test tube.

The sheet of paper is placed over the mouth of the tube, which is then inverted over one of the holes in the oiled silk and the paper slipped out of the way. When the leech has taken hold, the test tube is removed and the body of the leech is then left lying on the oiled silk. If the leech refuses to suck, it should be replaced in the tube while the skin is moistened with the sweetened milk. If it still refuses, then another leech should be tried.

Each leech is applied in the same way, and it will remain sucking for half to one hour. If it is desired to remove one before it has finished sucking, a little salt placed on the head will make it drop off. Leeches must never be pulled off. As they drop off they are placed in the bowl of phenol, but if they are likely to be used again, they should be placed in the bowl containing salt water and transferred to a container of cold water when they have vomited up the blood.

The bites are dressed with the circular pads firmly applied with adhesive plaster.

Occasionally leech-bites continue to bleed for a considerable time, and it may be necessary to apply a dressing of adrenaline in place of the dry dressing.

Liniments and Ointments

Liniments and ointments containing irritant substances are used for the relief of pain and stiffness.

In some cases the action of the liniment is assisted by fairly vigorously rubbing the area when applying it. In the case of tender, painful areas such as the swollen joints of the patient with rheumatoid arthritis or acute rheumatism rubbing should be avoided.

Liniments should be warmed before use.

Examples of such applications are:
  (1) Camphor liniment.
  (2) Methyl salicylate (oil of wintergreen) and menthol liniment.

Local Applications for Special Conditions.

Starch Poultice. This is used for the removal of scabs in skin diseases such as impetigo.

Requirements:

A sufficient quantity of powdered starch.
Boric powder.
Old linen cut to the required size.
Boiling water.
Cold water.
A board.

A mixing bowl.

A spoon.

A palette knife.

A small saucepan.

Jaconet or gutta-percha tissue for covering the poultice.

Bandages. If applied to the head, a cotton cap or a triangular bandage is convenient.

Measure the starch into the mixing bowl ($1\frac{1}{2}$ tablespoonfuls for every $\frac{1}{2}$ pint of water used will give the required consistency when cooked) and mix with it 1 teaspoonful of boric powder.

Break up the starch with sufficient cold water to make a thick paste, add the boiling water, and stir well until the starch turns clear. Pour the mixture into the saucepan and boil for two minutes.

Allow to cool slightly and then spread it evenly on the linen about $\frac{3}{4}$ inch thick.

When applied, the poultice should be almost cold and have the consistency of a jelly.

Cover with the protective material and bandage into position.

The application is left on for six to twelve hours.

When the poultice is taken off the scabs should be gently removed with dressing forceps and warm olive oil.

Unna's Paste. This application is a mixture of gelatin, glycerin and zinc powder. It is applied as a dressing and a support for varicose ulcers of the leg.

Requirements:

Unna's paste in a jar standing in hot water to melt it.

A large brush.

Open-wove cotton bandage or a gauze bandage.

A crêpe velpeau bandage.

The skin of the leg should be cleaned and the patient sits with the leg supported on a leg rest or a stool. The melted paste is applied with a brush thickly on to the skin and covered with a single layer of bandage applied smoothly, but tightly so that the paste oozes through. About six layers of paste and bandage are applied. When set, the dressing must be really tight. A supporting bandage of crêpe velpeau or elastic is applied over the dressing, which is usually left on for a week or longer.

"Viscopaste" bandages supplied ready for use have largely replaced Unna's paste as a supporting dressing.

Bisgard's Treatment for Varicose Ulcers

Bisgard's solution containing 1 per cent. aluminium acetate and 3 per cent. boric acid is applied as a wet dressing using twenty layers of gauze in order to ensure that the dressing is really wet. It is covered with a protective layer of oiled silk or non-absorbent wool. Wool padding is required behind the Achilles tendon of the heel and the lateral and medial malleoli. The leg is then firmly bandaged from the toes to the knee with an elastic webbing bandage. The patient is shown how to carry out the treatment at home. Each evening she removes the old dressing, massages the whole leg and the area around the ulcer before applying a fresh dressing which can be kept in place at night by a gauze bandage. In the morning a fresh dressing is applied and covered with the elastic webbing bandage which must be worn all day.

The patient is instructed to walk as much as possible but to avoid standing.

Cold Applications

The superficial application of cold depletes the circulation in the skin, relieving pressure and preventing swelling. It also causes increase of muscle tone.

It may be employed in the treatment of injuries of the soft tissues such as sprains, and in inflammatory conditions accompanied by congestion. It may also be used to arrest hæmorrhage. If the skin of the part becomes purple and discoloured, it is an indication that the application of cold should be discontinued.

Cold Compress. *Requirements:*

A double fold of white lint.
Iced water or lead lotion.
Jaconet.
Bandage.

The lint is wrung out of the iced water or lotion and applied to the part, covered with jaconet and a bandage. The application must be changed frequently, so that it is kept both moist and cold.

Evaporating Compress. *Requirements:*

    A dressing mackintosh.

    A double piece of white lint.

    Ice-cold water, or a mixture of equal parts of spirit and
        water.

    An open-wove bandage.

    A bed cradle.

The lint wrung out of the lotion is placed on the part, and
if necessary kept in position with a light bandage.   The lint
and bandage must be kept moist.

If the part being treated is a limb, a cradle should be placed
over it and the bedclothes arranged to give a free current of
air to resist evaporation.

Ice Bag. *Requirements:*

    Chipped ice.

    Ice pick.

    Salt.

    Ice bag.

    A flannel cover for the bag or a piece of lint.

    A bed cradle.

The bag is one-third filled with chipped ice to which 1 or
2 teaspoonfuls of salt have been added.   The air is expelled
and the bag carefully dried outside.

It is then placed in the flannel cover and suspended so that
it rests lightly on the skin.   For this purpose it is convenient
to suspend the bag from a cradle.

It must be refilled as soon as the ice has melted.

If an ice bag is not obtainable, a rubber sponge bag or a
polythene bag can be used as a substitute, but care must be
taken to suspend it in such a manner that it cannot leak.

Ice Poultice. This is sometimes found to be a useful
application as it is much lighter than the ice bag.

Requirements:

    Gutta-percha tissue.

    Wool.

    Salt.

    Chipped ice.

    Chloroform.

    A small paint brush.

    A piece of lint.

    Bandage.

A piece of gutta-percha tissue is cut to the required size, rather larger than twice the size of the finished poultice.

A thin layer of cotton wool ¼ inch smaller all round is placed on the tissue and one half of it covered with a thick layer of chipped ice and a sprinkling of salt. The other half of the wool and tissue is folded over the layer of ice. The poultice is finished by sealing the edges of the gutta-percha tissue with chloroform, using the paint brush.

The poultice should be changed as soon as the ice melts.

29

Methods of Treatment: Baths, Sponging, Packs

BATHS may be ordered for any of the following reasons:
- (1) To cleanse.
- (2) To stimulate the action of the skin.
- (3) To act as a sedative.
- (4) To reduce temperature.
- (5) To treat special conditions, as, for example, skin diseases.

Hot Baths

A hot bath at a temperature of 100° to 105° F. may be used for both its cleansing and sedative action. It will relieve pain due to muscular stiffness, and may also be ordered for the treatment of infantile convulsions or resuscitating the new-born infant.

It is particularly important to take the temperature of the bath for an infant or young child, as fatal scalds have occurred from neglecting this precaution.

The duration of the bath is from three to fifteen minutes.

A higher temperature (110° to 112° F.) is useful for relieving pain and stiffness following excessive muscular exertion, or in chronic rheumatic joint complaints, but care must be taken to prevent subsequent chilling.

If the hot bath is prolonged it is apt to have a depressing effect on the heart and circulatory system, owing to the dilatation of the superficial blood vessels, the muscular relaxation produced, and the interference of loss of heat from the body. The symptoms produced will be a rapid low-tension pulse, shallow rapid respirations, muscular weakness and faintness.

Medicated Baths

Mustard Bath. This may be ordered for its general stimulating effect, or to treat colds and chills.

4 to 6 oz. of mustard may be placed in a muslin bag, which is squeezed in the water, or it may be mixed to a paste with sufficient tepid water and added to the bath. The average full bath is 30 gallons.

Alkaline Baths. 4 to 6 oz. of sodium bicarbonate to 30 gallons of water. This may be ordered for the relief of irritation in skin conditions, or to aid the removal of crusts.

Saline Baths. Sterile normal saline baths may be used in the treatment of extensive burns. Hypertonic saline baths, 3 lb. of salt to 30 gallons of water may be ordered in the treatment of septic skin conditions.

Bran Bath. 2 lb. of bran to 30 gallons of water. This may be ordered as a soothing bath in eczematous skin conditions.

The bran should be tied in a muslin bag and placed in a large bowl. Boiling water is then poured over it, and when cool enough to handle the bag of bran is well squeezed and the fluid added to the bath. Oatmeal may be used in the same way in place of bran.

Starch Bath. 2 lb. of starch to 30 gallons of water. This may be used for the same conditions as a bran bath.

The starch is mixed to a paste with cold water, and then sufficient boiling water is poured on to make a mucilage. This is added to the warm water in the bath.

The duration of the treatment in the case of baths used for relief of skin conditions is usually ten to fifteen minutes.

Tepid Sponging

This form of treatment is employed in order to reduce temperature in febrile cases and is also useful for its sedative action. The reduction of temperature may not be more than two degrees, but the patient is usually much more comfortable after the treatment and will probably sleep.

Requirements:

A large washing bowl.

Jugs of hot and cold water.

A bath thermometer.

Small bowl with cold or iced water and compresses to apply to the head.

A hot-water bottle.

Soap, spirit and powder to give the necessary attention to the back and other pressure areas at the same time.

Two or more sponges or large pieces of lint. In cases where the temperature is very high the treatment is often more effective if additional sponges are used. One sponge is placed on the nape of the neck. one in each axilla, one in each hand, one behind each knee joint. These are changed as they become warm.

Towels.

Long mackintosh.

Two blankets.

The bed is stripped and the long mackintosh and blanket rolled under the patient. The nightgown is removed, leaving the patient covered with a blanket. The hot-water bottle is placed at the feet and the cold compress applied to the head.

The water for sponging should be between 80° and 90° F.

The face is first sponged and dried.

Using long sweeping strokes, one arm is sponged from the shoulder to the hand, using a fresh sponge as the one in use becomes warm. About three minutes is allowed for the sponging of each part.

As each part is finished it should be slightly dried and covered with the blanket. Some moisture should be left on the skin as the evaporation of this cools the body surface and helps to reduce the temperature. The water should be kept at the right temperature by the addition of hot or cold water as required.

The upper limbs, the chest and abdomen, and the lower limbs are all sponged in turn. The patient is then carefully turned over and the back sponged with long strokes from the neck to the buttocks. Pressure areas should receive attention while the patient is turned over, and then the under blanket and long mackintosh are rolled against the patient and the draw sheet arranged so that it can be drawn through. The patient is then rolled over to the opposite side and the long mackintosh and blanket removed.

The patient's gown is replaced and he is covered with a sheet and a light blanket. The cold compress is removed and the hair brushed. He should then be given a drink and left undisturbed.

The temperature is taken at the end of thirty minutes.

A cold sponge may be ordered, in which case the temperature of the water should be 60° to 65° F. An ice bag may be applied to the head in place of the compress.

If warm sponging is ordered, the temperature of the water used should be 110° to 115° F.

Hot Packs

In the past hot packs were ordered to promote sweating in cases of renal disease but most physicians consider that this treatment has no value in relieving œdema or in getting rid of toxins which the damaged kidneys are not able to deal with effectively.

Local hot packs may be used in the treatment of the acute stage of poliomyelitis. The effect of the application of heat to the affected muscles is to diminish pain and spasm and this allows passive and active movements to be carried out at an earlier stage than would otherwise be possible. The blood supply to the area is also improved. It is stated that an increase in the rate and depth of respiration may result.

Requirements:

Triangular pieces of blanket cut to the required size and stitched. The size will depend on the individual patient and the area to which the packs are to be applied, *e.g.* shoulders, hips, lower limb or trunk.

Triangular pieces of gamgee tissue and jaconet to cover the blanket.

A wringer of suitable size and sufficiently strong material, such as strong cotton ticking. If a wringing machine is available this will not be needed.

Triangular bandages.

Methods of heating the packs. The packs may be placed in the wringer in boiling water in a sterilizer or fish kettle.

Where the treatment is being carried out for a number of patients at frequent intervals a domestic washing machine with a wringer attached is very useful and there are also commercial "hot pack machines" made for this purpose. Another method is to use a water sterilizer, keeping the level of the water several inches below the perforated metal tray. The packs are placed in the tray over the boiling water and it is not necessary to wring them out before use.

The pieces of gamgee tissue used to cover the packs should be warmed before use. To prevent chilling during the application of the packs the patient is usually nursed between thin woollen or flannelette blankets. After heating by whichever method is used the packs are brought to the bed-side in between two warm bowls. If hand wringing is necessary this is done at the bedside.

After applying the pack it is covered with the piece of jaconet and the warmed gamgee tissue. The packs may be changed every ten minutes for half an hour then removed and the area covered with the gamgee tissue kept in place with a triangular bandage. The treatment is usually repeated every two hours at first and later the intervals may be lengthened to every four or every six hours.

The patient's condition should be carefully observed during the treatment. A rise of temperature or pulse rate or any sign of respiratory distress may necessitate terminating the procedure at least for the time being. Some patients may appreciate a cold compress applied to the forehead or a cool drink to sip. It is also essential that paralysed muscles are not subjected to any strain or stretching during the treatment.

The pieces of blanket need thorough drying after use either by hanging in the sun or in a suitable warm place such as a drying cupboard. They should be boiled for twenty minutes once a week. A blanket, if allowed to remain damp, is a very good growing ground for fungus.

30

First Aid and Treatment in Emergencies

FIRST aid is the temporary treatment given, in case of accident or emergency, pending the arrival of a doctor or the removal of the patient to hospital.

General Rules

Send for medical aid. A written message giving as much information as possible should be sent,

Treat the most serious condition first. These will be in order of urgency: cessation of breathing, profuse hæmorrhage, shock.

When treating an unconscious patient, keep him turned on to one side or prone, if possible, if not keep the head well turned to the side, lower than the trunk and make sure that the tongue is not obstructing the air-way. This will prevent saliva trickling down the trachea, an event which is likely to lead to pneumonia later. Do not try to give an unconscious patient or a patient who is vomiting anything by mouth.

Remember that if a patient is lying on the ground he will lose heat rapidly, and rugs should be placed under him as well as over him. If the patient is conscious reassure him as far as possible, and try to prevent would-be helpers from crowding round him and exciting him, or otherwise doing harm.

Shock

The term shock is used to denote the condition which is very liable to occur as a result of any serious injury, particularly if accompanied by severe loss of blood or plasma.

The important feature in shock is the reduction in the volume of the circulating blood and this may be due to actual loss of blood or plasma or to loss of tone in the blood vessels (vasovagal reaction) which means that a proportion of the available blood is temporarily out of circulation. The signs which are usually accepted as evidence of shock are pallor, cold skin, a weak quick pulse and low blood pressure. Thirst, sweating, restlessness, dyspnœa and vomiting are some of the general signs and symptoms that the patient may exhibit.

Treatment. If the patient is bleeding immediate steps must be taken to stop the blood loss. Effective treatment of circulatory failure due to hæmorrhage can be carried out only by transfusion and therefore the patient must be removed to hospital without delay. General measures which can be applied as first aid are rest, reassurance and conservation of body heat. The patient should be lying down in as comfortable a position as possible. Restlessness may be due, at least in part to fear and anxiety, therefore every effort should be made to encourage the injured person to feel that he is safe and that competent treatment is being and will be given. A certain amount of warmth is comforting and this can be supplied by warm blankets and clothing, but overheating is harmful since it causes dilatation of the surface vessels, tends to produce sweating and a further fall in blood pressure. If the patient's clothing is wet it should be removed if it is possible to do this without causing him further harm, the first aider should remember that extreme gentleness is necessary in handling the patient as any movement is likely to cause pain, increase shock and possibly increase bleeding.

It is wise in most circumstances to withhold fluids by mouth as an anæsthetic may be required when the patient is admitted to hospital. This should, however not be regarded as a hard and fast rule as there may be occasions when common sense dictates that fluids such as tea or coffee should be given unless the patient is vomiting or there are signs of abdominal injury, as for example in circumstances where there is likely to be long delay in obtaining medical treatment or transporting the patient to hospital.

Hæmorrhage
[Escape of Blood from the Blood Vessels]

Causes. (1) Injury to the blood vessel walls as a result of an accidental wound, or during an operation.

(2) Diseases of the vessel walls—*e.g.* an aneurysm dilating

and thinning the wall. Malignant growths, ulcers, or suppurating wounds are also conditions which may lead to rupture of the vessel walls.

(3) Diseases of the blood, as for example hæmophilia in which the blood is deficient in clotting power.

Types of Hæmorrhage

(1) *Classed according to the Type of Vessel Injured.*

(a) **Arterial Hæmorrhage.** The blood is bright red and escapes in spurts. If a large artery is damaged the force behind the escape of blood is great, and this is the most difficult type of hæmorrhage to control.

(b) **Venous Hæmorrhage.** The blood is dark in colour and pours out in a steady stream. If a large vein is injured the loss will be rapid, but the pressure in the veins is almost nil and the bleeding can be easily controlled.

(c) **Capillary Hæmorrhage.** There is a general oozing, easily controlled from the wound.

(2) *Classed according to the Time at which it Occurs.*

(a) **Primary.** Occurring at the time of the injury. The amount will be influenced by the type of injury, as well as by the type of vessel damaged. Clean-cut wounds with a sharp instrument are likely to bleed freely; lacerated wounds will bleed less, as the blood clots more quickly with this type of injury.

(b) **Reactionary Hæmorrhage.** Occurring within twenty-four hours of the injury or operation, and after the cessation of the primary hæmorrhage. It is likely to occur during the recovery period, when the blood pressure is rising, in patients who have suffered a severe degree of shock.

(c) **Secondary Hæmorrhage.** This results from sepsis destroying the vessel wall and occurs after twenty-four hours and within fourteen days of the injury. Although rarely seen in present day hospital practice this possibility should always be kept in mind when dealing with infected wounds.

(3) *Classed according to the Site of the Hæmorrhage.*

(a) **External Hæmorrhage.** Bleeding from a visible site, such as a wound.

13+

(b) **Internal Hæmorrhage.** Bleeding taking place into one
of the body cavities, such as the peritoneal cavity.
Such a hæmorrhage may also be described as a
concealed hæmorrhage, or if the blood escapes from
one of the natural orifices of the body it may then
be described as an internal revealed hæmorrhage.

Signs and Symptoms of Severe Loss of Blood. Increasing
pallor of the skin and mucous membranes; a low temperature;
deep sighing respirations; restlessness and anxiety; increasingly rapid pulse; thirst; a feeling of faintness, blurred vision
and gradual loss of consciousness. Unless the hæmorrhage
is concealed, there will be visible blood.

Natural Arrest of Hæmorrhage. This is achieved by:

(1) Contraction of the severed vessel walls and retraction
of the inner coat, causing a diminution of the bore of the
vessel.

(2) Clotting of the blood, sealing the cut ends of the vessel.

(3) Lowering of the blood pressure, reducing the force of
the circulation, accompanied by a feeling of faintness which
aids nature by ensuring that the patient assumes a recumbent
position and so further reduces the blood pressure.

Treatment of Hæmorrhage

Send for medical aid. Place the patient lying flat with
the head low, unless the bleeding is from the head or neck.
If the bleeding is from a limb, elevate the part.

Apply direct pressure to the bleeding part. If nothing is
to hand and the bleeding is profuse, the operator's thumbs
may be placed on the wound, pressing firmly. A pad and
bandage should be obtained as soon as possible.

If pressure on the wound does not stop the bleeding from
a cut artery, apply pressure over the artery at the appropriate
pressure point.

Apply a tourniquet if the bleeding is still not controlled
and the part will allow of such a procedure—*i.e.* if the injury
is to a limb.

Ensure a plentiful supply of fresh air for the patient and
keep him warm.

When the bleeding is controlled, give fluids.

Keep a careful watch for recurrence.

Pressure points may be found in certain sites where an
artery is superficial and lies over a bone.

The artery should be compressed between the operator's thumbs and the underlying bone.

The brachial artery may be compressed against the inner side of the humerus about midway between the axilla and the elbow.

The ulnar and radial arteries may be compressed against the underlying ulna and radius by pressure of both thumbs just above the wrist. Acute flexion of the elbow over a pad in the bend of the elbow is a method which is easy to use and often successful.

The femoral artery may be compressed against the pelvis midway between the symphysis pubis and the anterior superior iliac spine.

The subclavian artery may, though with considerable difficulty be compressed against the first rib behind the clavicle.

The carotid artery may be compressed against the transverse process of the sixth cervical vertebra at the level of the cricoid cartilage.

The temporal artery in front of the ear just above the external auditory meatus may be compressed against the zygomatic process of the temporal bone.

The popliteal artery may be compressed by placing a firm pad in the popliteal space and acutely flexing the knee.

Tourniquets. Application of digital pressure over the main artery and pressure on the wound are likely to be successful in the majority of cases; where a main artery is damaged, however, it may not be possible to maintain the digital pressure for a sufficient length of time to control the bleeding until the patient can have medical attention. An improvised tourniquet may then be applied.

A piece of lint, a layer of clothing or any available material should be placed between the tourniquet and the skin.

The tourniquet should be gently released at the end of fifteen minutes, it should be left in position but not tightened again unless bleeding recommences.

A tourniquet should not be used unless other methods of arresting severe hæmorrhage fail. If not efficiently applied a tourniquet may fail to compress the main artery but will occlude the veins and so increase the bleeding; if it is applied with sufficient pressure to be effective it must be remembered that a tourniquet will cut off the entire blood supply to the area distal to the tourniquet and therefore ischæmic paralysis of the muscles or even gangrene of the limb are possible consequences. If when the patient is first seen a tourniquet is found to have been used and there is no note of the time of application it should be cautiously released and not reapplied unless there is a recurrence of uncontrollable hæmorrhage.

Special Types of Hæmorrhage

Hæmorrhage from a Varicose Vein. This may be very profuse, but is easily controlled. Firm pressure should be applied to the site of the hæmorrhage and the leg elevated.

Hæmorrhage in the Alimentary Tract. Vomiting of blood (hæmatemesis). The blood is dark in colour and acid in reaction.

While awaiting medical aid, the patient should receive the general treatment for hæmorrhage. He should be reassured and told that he will help himself greatly if he will lie as still as possible. Nothing should be given by mouth.

When bleeding occurs in the upper part of the alimentary tract a large stool of a tarry colour and consistency may be passed (melæna). The first-aid treatment is the same as that for hæmatemesis.

Bright red blood passed per rectum is most commonly due to piles, but also occurs in cancer of the rectum. The bleeding is seldom severe enough to require first-aid treatment, but the patient should be advised to consult a doctor so that the cause may be investigated.

Hæmoptysis. Coughing of blood from the lungs. The blood is bright red and frothy. The patient should be supported in a comfortable position, sitting up. He should be reassured, told that the bleeding will stop and asked to cough up the blood, but without straining.

Epistaxis. Bleeding from the nose. The patient should sit upright and a sponge of cold water or ice may be held on the bridge of the nose. Direct pressure on the nostril on the bleeding side may be effectual. If the bleeding is severe and not easily arrested, medical aid must be obtained.

Cerebral Hæmorrhage. This may be caused by injury or disease of the blood vessels. The symptoms and signs that result from such a cerebral catastrophe are due to pressure within the skull on the brain tissue. The first aid treatment

Simple, Compound, Commuted, Greenstick,
Depressed, Spiral. Impact.

of a patient who becomes unconscious as a result of cerebral
hæmorrhage is the same as that described for a patient with a
severe head injury on page 323.

Fractures

The word fracture quite simply means a break, in medical
terms it is used to describe a break in a bone.

The two important classes of fractures are:

(1) Simple, or closed, in which there is no communica-
tion between the broken bone and the external air.

(2) Compound, or open, in which the fracture communicates with the external air, either through
the skin or a mucous surface.

The aim to be borne in mind in treating a simple fracture
is to prevent that fracture from becoming compound.

The first consideration in treating a compound fracture
is to get the patient to hospital as quickly as possible.

Signs and Symptoms of a Fracture (not necessarily all
present):

Faystory   Deformity

Pain.

Tenderness immediately over the site of the break.

Swelling and bruising.

Loss of function.

Unnatural mobility.

Crepitus, or grating of the broken ends of the bone.

Shock, varying with the degree of injury and the type
of patient; it is likely to be present and marked in
elderly patients, and in fractures inflicted with
considerable violence or accompanied by injuries to
other structures.

The history of the accident may be helpful.

The nurse should not attempt to elicit the signs of unnatural
mobility or crepitus.

General Principles of Treatment. (1) The patient should
be kept lying down, unless the particular injury makes this
an unsuitable position.

(2) The patient should be treated for shock.

(3) Any open wound should be covered with as clean a
dressing as can be obtained.

(4) Padded splints should be applied to immobilize the
fractured ends of the bone. The splints should be wide

enough, long enough and strong enough to keep the joint above and the joint below the fracture at rest.

(5) Safe transport for the patient should be arranged as quickly as possible. Fractures of the lower extremity, pelvis spine or skull should be transported on a stretcher.

Splints may be improvised from pieces of wood, such as packing cases, sticks, umbrellas or from stout cardboard. They may be padded with any material to hand (thick woollen stuffs, cotton wool or newspaper). They may be secured by handkerchiefs, towels, belts, or any available material in the absence of bandages. The upper extremity can often be splinted by bandaging the arm to the patient's body and the lower limb may be bandaged to the undamaged leg. If the leg is the site of a suspected fracture, on no account should the patient be allowed to stand.

If the forearm is injured, a sling should be used; if the upper arm, then the arm may be bandaged to the trunk.

Bandages should be just sufficiently firmly applied to keep the splints in position; they should not be too tight, as the injured limb is likely to swell and the blood supply may be impeded.

A stretcher may be improvised from a door, a hurdle or a gate or a strong rug may be tied by the corners to broom handles and a stick placed transversely at either end.

Special Fractures

(1) **Ribs.** The special danger of a broken rib is that the ends of the bone may damage the lung. Following the injury the patient may complain of great pain on breathing and may cough up blood.

It is essential that medical aid should be sought early, as chest complications are apt to occur especially in elderly patients.

The first-aid treatment consists of supporting the patient in the most comfortable position—which is usually sitting up—applying a binder round the chest at the end of expiration to restrict the movements of the chest wall, and keeping the patient warm.

(2) **Spine.** If there is reason to suspect that a patient has a fractured spine, he should be kept lying still and treated for shock until sufficient help is at hand to lift him carefully on to a stretcher and convey him to hospital. It is important

not to bend or twist the spinal column when moving the patient. The best position in which to transport him is lying on his back with small pillows or pads under the hollow of the neck, the small of the back and below the calves of the legs.

(3) **Pelvis.** Fractures of the pelvis may injure the bladder, urethra or rectum. The patient should have a firm binder round the pelvis for support and should be lifted, without rolling, on to the stretcher. Bearing in mind the possible injury to the urethra, the patient should be warned not to pass urine.

(4) **Femur.** The best first-aid treatment is the application of traction by means of a Thomas's splint. The splint is applied over the clothing, and extension made by taking a clove hitch round the foot and ankle and fastening the ends of the bandage to the end of the splint. The limb is supported in the splint by means of broad fold bandages or strips of flannel. Two pieces of Gooch's splinting or stiff corrugated cardboard should be placed on the front and back of the thigh for added support. A piece of wood or a skewer is placed between the two tails of the hitch and used as a windlass to tighten the extension. (See p. 171.)

(5) **Skull.** Any injury to the head which produces unconsciousness, however short in duration, must be considered serious, and the patient on recovery should be advised not to continue with what he was doing at the time of the accident, but should be taken to a doctor or hospital.

Following a severe head injury the patient is likely to be deeply unconscious, he may be bleeding from the nose, mouth and ears, or into the orbit. If the fracture has torn the membranes covering the brain and communicates with the nose or the ear, there may be a steady and continuous leaking of clear fluid, the cerebrospinal fluid. There may be twitching of the muscles of one side of the body, convulsions, paralysis of one side, and the patient may have incontinence of urine or fæces.

The patient must be taken to hospital as soon as possible. Any external wound should be covered with a clean dressing. False teeth and spectacles should be removed. The head should be kept to one side to allow blood and saliva to run out of the mouth and to keep the air-way clear. If fluid or blood is escaping from the external auditory meatus a clean dressing should be applied, no attempt to mop out or syringe the ears should be made. Tight clothing should be loosened.

Dislocations

A dislocation is a displacement of the joint surfaces of two or more bones as a result of injury. At the same time the soft structures surrounding the joint are damaged.

Signs and Symptoms: (1) Deformity; (2) loss of movement; (3) pain; (4) swelling.

The shoulder-joint is fairly easily dislocated, the fingers, jaw, ankle and elbow joints may also be dislocated without great violence but considerable force is required to produce a dislocation of the hip joint.

Treatment. Support the limb in as comfortable a position as possible with bandages or a sling. A dislocation is most easily reduced immediately after the injury, therefore no time should be lost in getting the patient to a doctor. In certain circumstances it may be necessary to reduce a dislocation of the jaw without medical aid. The patient should be seated facing the operator, who places her thumbs on the back lower teeth and then presses downwards and backwards. Some protection, such as several layers of bandage or handkerchiefs, should be wound round the thumbs, which should be removed quickly from the patient's mouth, as the jaw will snap into place suddenly. After this procedure a jaw bandage should be applied for support. (See pp. 163, 165).

Sprains

A sprain is an injury to the soft tissues of a joint involving the muscles and ligaments. The usual situations are the ankle, wrist and thumb.

Signs and Symptoms: (1) Pain; (2) swelling; (3) discolouration.

Treatment. The possibility of a dislocation or a fracture should be considered and the patient urged to get medical attention. In the meantime he should not use the limb and some support may be given by the application of a firm bandage. Elevation of the part and cold applications may help to prevent swelling. If there is already much swelling and bruising, hot applications will probably give most relief.

Burns and Scalds

A burn is an injury produced by dry heat, and a scald by

moist heat. From the point of view of first aid the immediate results of the injury and the treatment are the same. Burns are likely immediately to endanger life as a result of shock, later as a result of toxæmia, or severe sepsis. It should be understood that the patient's life is in danger from an extensive burn, even if it be entirely superficial; if one quarter of the total skin surface is involved the injury is extremely serious.

Medical aid should be obtained as speedily as possible. Full treatment of the burnt area will be carried out only in hospital, but morphine may be required immediately for the relief of pain. The patient should be moved as little as possible and gentle handling is essential. A burnt patient may complain of thirst and small amounts of water may be given to relieve this. It is better to give small quantities frequently rather than to encourage the patient to drink large amounts as vomiting is not unusual.

The burnt area, if exposed, should be covered with the cleanest dressing to hand, if sterile dressings are not available clean towels or sheets may be used as substitutes, the surface which has been folded in, and therefore protected from dust should be placed next to the burnt skin. Blankets and rugs should not be allowed to come in contact with an exposed burnt area as they are potential sources of heavy bacterial contamination. If the injured area is covered by clothing this is best left undisturbed.

Where burns are likely to be common accidental injuries, as for instance in certain industries, the use of a water-soluble cream containing penicillin or sulphonamide and 1 per cent. cetrimide is one of the dressings recommended for use in first aid. Any first-aid dressing should be carried out with all the aseptic precautions that the circumstances permit. The dresser should wash her hands and dry them on a clean towel before handling any dressing material and an improvised mask, *e.g.* a clean pocket handkerchief, should be worn.

Scalds of the Throat and Mouth. Such accidents are not uncommon in young children, who may suck the spout of a teapot or boiling kettle.

Medical aid should be obtained at once; swelling of the upper air passages may cause obstruction of the air way and tracheostomy may be necessary. The child should be put to bed and kept warm. Fomentations may be applied to the neck and sips of olive oil given by mouth.

13*

Chemical Burns. The chemical should be thoroughly washed off with warm water. If the nature of the substance is known, a neutralizing agent may be used—*e.g.* a corrosive acid such as nitric acid should be washed off with a solution of sodium bicarbonate or lime water. Strong lysol or carbolic acid splashed on the skin is best removed with surgical spirit or methylated spirit. Caustic soda burns may be treated with a weak acid such as vinegar.

Chemical Burns of the Eye. The eye should be opened (an assistant may be needed to do this) and then thoroughly washed out with clean water for at least fifteen minutes. The eye is then covered with a pad and bandage. Medical treatment is essential and urgent in order to prevent permanent damage.

Poisons

Classes of Poisons. (1) Corrosive substances—*e.g.* strong acids or alkalis, strong lysol or carbolic acid.

(2) Irritants—*e.g.* mercuric and arsenical preparations, food poisoning.

(3) Substances acting on the central nervous system—*e.g.* narcotics (opium) or convulsants (strychnine).

Medical aid should be obtained at once and as much information given as possible. Any bottles or containers likely to have held the poison should be saved, as also should the vomit or excreta of the patient.

Aims of Treatment:

To remove the poison.
To neutralize the poison.
To combat the effects of the poison.

To remove a poison which has been swallowed an emetic should be given at once; this should be followed by a stomach wash-out. The contra-indications to an emetic are signs of burning round the mouth and lips, indicating that the poison is corrosive. A stomach wash-out will probably be given by the doctor after neutralization of the poison.

Simple emetics likely to be at hand are:

(1) Salt and water, 2 tablespoonfuls to ½ pint of warm water.

(2) Mustard and water, 1 tablespoonful to ½ pint of warm water.

(3) Copious drinks of tepid water.

Mechanical stimulation by tickling the back of the throat may be successful.

To neutralize the effect of the poison the appropriate antidote, if known and available, should be given.

A chemical antidote is one which neutralizes the poison by altering its chemical composition—*e.g.* the use of an acid to neutralize an alkali.

A physiological antidote is one which has the opposite effect on the body from that of the poison—*e.g.* strong coffee is a physiological antidote to narcotic poisons, sedative drugs such as bromide are antidotes to the convulsant poisons.

To combat the effects of the poison the symptoms of pain and shock should be treated, when present. Respiratory failure should be treated by respiratory stimulants such as inhalations of smelling salts or ammonia, or by artificial respiration. If available, oxygen and carbon dioxide should be administered. Damage to tissues by swallowed corrosive poisons should be treated by giving demulcents.

Demulcents likely to be at hand are: milk, white of egg, starch or cornflour mucilage, gruel. Milk and white of egg are particularly useful in poisoning by acid substances, as they have the power of "buffering" or sopping up acids.

Loss of Consciousness

Loss of consciousness may be due to a temporary depletion of blood in the brain, as is the case in the simple fainting attack, or to actual loss of blood, as in hæmorrhage, or may occur in various serious conditions such as cerebral hæmorrhage, poisoning, asphyxia, heart disease, kidney disease and diabetes.

A simple fainting attack is usually the result of prolonged standing, especially in a hot and stuffy atmosphere, or may be due to emotional causes such as an unpleasant sight (*e.g.* a street accident), or to fatigue or hunger.

Signs and Symptoms:

Pallor.

Restlessness.

Perspiration round the mouth and on the forehead.

EXAMPLES OF TYPES OF POISONS, SYMPTOMS PRODUCED AND APPROPRIATE FIRST-AID TREATMENT

Poison	Signs and Symptoms	Treatment
1. *Corrosive poisons, e.g.* phenol or dipol.	Burns on lips and mouth. Intense pain from mouth to stomach. Vomiting. Marked shock.	Immediate treatment, dilute the poison by giving tap water or milk if the patient can swallow. If the poison is a coal tar disinfectant, a stomach wash out, using 1 per cent solution of Magnesium Sulphate (Epsom Salts), should be prepared; 2 fl. ozs. of liquid paraffin may be put down the tube after the wash-out.
2. *Irritant poisons, e.g.* Mercury preparations, arsenic.	Pain in abdomen. Vomiting; the vomit may contain blood and mucus. Diarrhœa. Collapse	Give an emetic, prepare for stomach wash-out. Treat collapse by warmth and hot applications to abdomen. Following the emetic or wash-out a demulcent mixture of milk and egg may be given.
3. *Poisons acting on the nervous system:* Hypnotic and Narcotic poisons, *e.g.* Morphine barbiturates.	Drowsiness, coma, slow respirations.	If the poison has been swallowed, give an emetic. Prepare for stomach wash-out. Stimulate patient by giving strong coffee, inhalation of smelling salts or ammonia. Artificial respiration if necessary. The specific antidote to opium or morphine is Nalorphine which combats respiratory failure. Drugs used to combat the effect of barbiturates include Nikethamide, Methedrine and Megimide.
Convulsant poisons, *e.g.* Strychnine	Restlessness, delirium, convulsions.	Emetic and stomach wash-out, if seen early. If patient is having convulsions, keep as quiet as possible. Drugs used to combat the convulsive poisons include anæsthetics such as Sodium Thiopentone and muscle relaxants, *e.g.* Tubocurarine, Scoline.

A feeling of nausea and faintness.

The patient becomes unsteady and falls to the ground.

The pulse is feeble and slow.

Treatment. If recognized before consciousness is lost, the patient should sit down with the head between the knees. When the feeling of faintness has passed he should lie flat in the fresh air for a short while.

If the patient has lost consciousness, he should be allowed to lie flat where he is and all tight clothing should be loosened. When he comes round he should rest for a while and be given a drink of water, sal volatile, or hot tea or coffee.

If a patient does not recover quickly from a fainting attack he should be kept at rest and medical aid obtained. The pulse should be noted; a quick feeble pulse may be the indication of a concealed hæmorrhage.

Convulsions

A convulsion is a series of involuntary contractions of the muscles during which the patient may or may not be unconscious.

Some of the causes of fits are epilepsy, hysteria, diseases or injuries of the brain and toxic conditions such as uræmia or eclampsia. In infants minor ailments or disturbances may cause the particular variety of fit known as an infantile convulsion.

An Epileptic Fit is characterized by the fact that the patient is unconscious and that the fit proceeds through certain definite stages. It may be preceded by a warning, or aura, which is a sensory disturbance peculiar to the particular patient. The aura may be a vague feeling of discomfort, a flash of light before the eyes, or a sensation of dizziness. The aura may give the patient sufficient time to lie down before the fit begins.

The first stage of the fit observed by the onlooker is the tonic stage. The patient commonly gives a cry and falls to the ground unconscious. The muscles are rigid, respiratory movements cease, he becomes blue in the face and the eyes are turned upwards. This stage lasts about thirty seconds.

He then passes into the clonic or convulsive stage. The rigidity of the muscles passes off, to be succeeded by violent

movements. The tongue is protruded and withdrawn, the
patient foams at the mouth and may be incontinent. This
stage lasts about sixty seconds.

Following the clonic stage, the patient passes into the
stage of coma, often followed by sleep.

Treatment. Unless the patient falls in such a situation
that he is in danger of injury, as, for example, close to a fire,
nothing need be done in the tonic stage except to loosen
any tight clothing. At the beginning of the clonic stage a
gag should be slipped into the mouth to prevent the tongue
from being bitten. This may be any suitable object to hand,
such as a piece of wood with a handkerchief wrapped round
one end. The movements of the limbs need not be restrained,
unless necessary to prevent the patient from hurting himself
on surrounding objects. When the fit is over the patient
should be allowed to rest. When he wakes up he will not
remember having had the fit, but if subject to epilepsy will
give a history of previous fits.

If the patient is known to have epileptic fits he may be
allowed to go home, but should be accompanied by a friend,
as it is possible that he may perform peculiar automatic
actions for which he is not responsible in his post-epileptic
state.

If there is doubt concerning the nature of the fit, or if the
patient has successive fits, medical aid should be obtained.

This type of epilepsy is known as major epilepsy, or grand
mal. The disease known as minor epilepsy, or petit mal, is
characterized by momentary loss of consciousness without
convulsive movements. No first-aid treatment is required,
but the patient should be accompanied to his home, as the
condition of post-epileptic automatism may also follow these
minor attacks.

Any other type of fit accompanied by convulsive movements requires the same first-aid treatment to prevent injury
to the patient, but medical aid should be sent for.

Hysterical Fit. Hysteria may show itself in many forms.
The hysterical fit is most commonly seen in young women
and may simulate in some ways the epileptic fit. The
muscles may be held rigid at first and then violent jerky
movements follow, but there are no definite stages. The
patient will not, as a rule, fall in such a manner as to hurt
herself, nor will the fit occur while she is alone. She is not

unconscious, although she is unlikely to take any apparent notice of her surroundings and will appear not to remember the circumstances of the fit afterwards. She will not bite her tongue, but may bite her lips or fingers. There is no incontinence of urine or fæces.

Treatment. The patient should be left quietly alone; all onlookers, especially sympathetic relations, should be asked to go away. The removal of the audience usually brings the fit to an end.

The subsequent treatment of the patient and investigation of the underlying cause of the condition are matters for the doctor.

Infantile Convulsions. Infantile convulsions were comparatively frequently seen when rickets was a common disease of childhood. Convulsions may also accompany the onset of a febrile illness in infancy. The immediate treatment is to place the infant in a warm cot in a quiet room. A doctor should see the infant, as the cause of the fit must be investigated.

Asphyxia

This is a condition in which there is interference with the normal exchange of gases between the atmospheric air and the body tissues.

Causes. (1) Obstruction to the air passages, as in strangulation, or inspiration of a foreign body.

(2) Drowning, pulmonary œdema.

(3) Poisonous gases, *e.g.* coal gas (carbon monoxide).

(4) Paralysis of the respiratory muscles.

(5) Depression of the respiratory centre in the brain as for example may be produced by an overdose of barbiturates or morphine.

Treatment. Send urgently for medical aid.

Attempt to remove the cause of the asphyxia, make sure that the airway is clear and carry out artificial respiration at once if breathing has ceased.

Artificial Respiration. One method of artificial respiration which has been in use for many years is Schäfer's method. The patient is placed prone on the ground with the head on one side and a pillow or folded coat under the upper part of the abdomen.

The operator kneels at the side of the patient, placing his

hands with the fingers lying together on the patient's back over the lower ribs and the thumbs parallel to the vertebral column. Swinging forwards, the chest is compressed; swinging back, the weight is taken off the hands allowing the chest to expand. These movements should be repeated about sixteen times per minute.

When the patient starts to breathe naturally he must be watched carefully, as respiration may cease again after a short time.

The advantages are that the position of the patient prevents obstruction to the airway from the tongue falling back, allows fluid to run out of the mouth, and at the same time helps by massaging the heart. It is also easier for the operator, and as the procedure may have to be carried on for a considerable time this is of importance.

The Holger-Nielsen method* introduced in Denmark has been recommended by the British Red Cross Society as their method of choice in artificial respiration. The essential movements of pressing and arm raising not only ventilate the lungs but stimulate the heart.

(1) *Immediate Action.* Carry the patient quickly to a smooth flat place. Peel off tight or heavy clothing and loosen tight articles such as the collar and belt. In cases of drowning, clear the mouth of mud, sea-weed, etc., with the forefinger wrapped in a handkerchief.

(2) *Turn the Patient.* If he is lying on his back, turn the patient into the prone position (*i.e.* face downwards) as follows: kneel on the right knee in front of his head with the left foot on the ground out to the side; arrange the centre of the body slightly to the right of that of the patient. Pull the patient's arms over his head.

Using both hands, grasp the patient's left arm, turning him over with a steady pull. As he comes on to his side, release the right hand and place it for the remainder of the turn under his forehead to prevent his face from striking the ground.

(3) *Arrange Position of Patient.* Arrange the patient's forehead on the support made by placing his hands one on top of the other. Make certain that his mouth and nose

* By courtesy of the Royal Life Saving Society, 14 Devonshire Street, London, W.1.

are completely unobstructed. If his mouth sinks towards the ground, raise his forehead an inch or so by placing the edge of a garment (*i.e.* a coat collar) under the hands. If necessary, turn the head slightly to one side.

(4) *Prepare for Artificial Respiration.* (*a*) Using the flat of the hand—wrist relaxed—slap the patient smartly once or twice between his shoulders. This usually causes the mouth to open, the tongue to fall forward, and, in drowning, to drive water out of the upper respiratory passages. If later it is found that the tongue is obstructing the passage of air, it must be drawn forward so that its tip protrudes slightly beyond the teeth.

(*b*) Place one knee 6–12 inches from the top of the patient's head, the inner side of the knee being in a straight line with the patient's cheek on the same side. Advance the other foot to the patient's elbow so that the heel is level with it and the toes point forward.

(*c*) Place both hands on the patient's back with the palms resting on the shoulder-blades, the thumbs on the spine, and the fingers pointing towards the feet (Fig. 62A).

(5) *Produce Expiration* (pressure). Without bending the elbows and using no force whatever, rock the trunk gently forward on to the straight arms until they are vertical, thus exerting a smooth, gentle, evenly increasing pressure from above downwards on to the patient's back.

This movement should take 2 seconds, estimated by slowly counting—one, two, three (Fig. 62B).

(6) *Induce Inspiration* (arm raising). (*a*) Counting four rock the trunk back allowing the hands to glide past the patient's shoulders until they can grasp his arms above the elbows.

(*b*) Using the straight arms, perform a steady, quick raising and pulling motion on the arms lasting 2 seconds, estimated by slowly counting—five, six, seven. Rock backwards a little, thus raising the patient's elbows to the level of his shoulders (Fig. 62C).

This action relieves the patient's chest of the weight of his trunk and lets the chest expand for a deep breath. The trunk itself must not be raised nor must the position of the hands be disturbed.

(7) *Continue Movements.* On the count of eight, lower the arms to the ground and move the hands to the initial

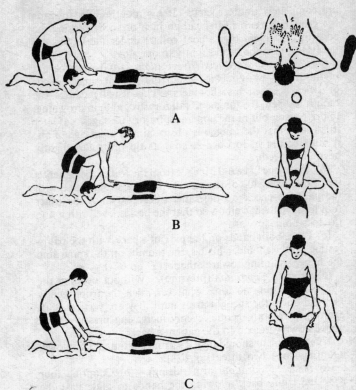

A

B

C

FIG. 62.—THE HOLGER-NIELSEN METHOD OF ARTIFICIAL RESPIRATION.

expiration position in 1 second. Continue at the rate of 9 complete respirations per minute.

(8) *Signs of Recovery.* When quivering of the body, a gasp, improved colour and movements of the patient show commencing recovery, continue artificial respiration until the improvement is established. Then continue with the arm-raising movement only, taking 2 seconds over each action of inspiration and expiration with no pause between them, *i.e.* 10 to 12 full respirations a minute.

If artificial respiration has to be continued for a prolonged time, change position periodically, *i.e.* kneel on the opposite knee, or transfer to another first-aider without interrupting the movements.

Artificial respiration should be carried on until the patient breathes naturally or until a doctor has stated that the patient is dead. If the heart is still beating, there is hope that the patient may recover if artificial respiration is kept up.

At the same time other helpers should be directed to procure warm dry clothing and a warm bed prepared for the patient when he can be moved, or arrangements made to take him to hospital. Chest complications are very liable to follow.

Mechanical Respirators

If artificial aid is likely to be required over a long period, as in respiratory paralysis, some form of mechanical apparatus is used. The aim in all the various types of apparatus is to produce regular changes in pressure either on the lungs or inside the lungs in order that ventilation of the lungs may be maintained.

The three main types of apparatus are:

Negative-positive apparatus where negative pressure applied to the chest wall causes inspiration and expiration is produced by a slight degree of positive pressure.

Positive pressure apparatus where pressure is applied to the chest and inspiration is brought about by elastic recoil when the pressure is released.

Positive pressure through the airway, either by means of a face mask, an endotracheal tube or through a tracheostomy tube.

Negative-positive Pressure

The Drinker and the Both respirator and modifications of these consist of a steel cabinet in which the patient's body is totally enclosed except for his head. An airtight seal is provided by means of a sponge rubber collar which fits round the neck. When the patient needs attention while in the cabinet there are portholes through which the nurse can insert her arms, also one large enough for the insertion of a bedpan, and these are provided with a seal in the form of a rubber cuff. The cabinet can be tilted so that accumulation of secretions in the mouth and pharynx can be prevented by

postural drainage. The pressure inside the cabinet is inter-
mittently and rhythmically altered by an electrically driven
pump, attached to the foot end of the cabinet by a length of
unkinkable rubber hose pipe. The main disadvantage of
this type of respirator is that nursing procedures are difficult
to carry out. However, if the patient can continue breathing
for short periods without the respirator, the bed on which
he lies can be withdrawn from the cabinet and the necessary
nursing attention can then be more efficiently given. If
necessary the patient can be kept breathing by using anæsthetic apparatus for a short period. Provision must be made
for the pump to be operated by hand in the event of a power
failure. A handle is supplied which can be attached to a
lever allowing manual operation to be brought into use in a
few seconds should the motor fail. It is most important
that nurses responsible for the care of a patient in a respirator
should be familiar with the procedure of attaching the handle
to the pump lever. Variations in the speed of the motor
are possible, thus allowing for adjustment of the respiratory
rate.

Positive Pressure to the Chest

An example of this type of apparatus is the Bragg-Paul
respirator which consists essentially of an inflatable bag
connected to a pump operated by an electric motor. The bag
is fastened round the patient's chest and slightly inflated.
The pressure in the bag is then alternately increased and
decreased by the action of the pump. This apparatus is
simple and can be worn when the patient is sitting up in a
chair. Its chief use is to assist the patient who has some
degree of movement in his respiratory muscles; it is not
sufficient where paralysis is complete.

Positive Pressure through the Airway

The principle on which these resuscitators and respirators
work is that the lungs are inflated by forcing air into the
air passages.

The Oxford resuscitator and various modifications of it
are used for resuscitation over a short period. A regulating
valve is attached to an oxygen cylinder connected to a rubber
facepiece. The facepiece is fitted with a hand-controlled
spring valve. When the spring is closed there is no escape of
oxygen to the atmosphere and the gas is forced into the lungs.

When the spring is released the flow of oxygen from the cylinder is cut off and the lungs are deflated by their own natural recoil.

The Beaver type of positive pressure apparatus. This is particularly useful when controlled respiration is required over a long period, as in the bulbospinal type of poliomyelitis, where respiratory paralysis is associated with paralysis of the pharynx and swallowing muscles.

A tracheostomy is performed and a cuffed rubber tube passed into the trachea. When the cuff is inflated the pharynx, nose and mouth are cut off from the rest of the respiratory tract and the secretions which the patient cannot swallow or expectorate can no longer enter the lungs. The tube is attached via an expiratory valve to a bellows type breathing bag which is alternately inflated and deflated by a small electrically driven motor. There is usually no need to supplement the oxygen in the normal room air in which the patient is being nursed, but if necessary oxygen can be added. Frequent suction is needed to keep the mouth and pharynx from "pooling" mucus and saliva. Feeding in these cases is carried out by means of an œsophageal tube passed through the nose into the stomach.

Treatment for Carbon Monoxide Poisoning. The patient should be removed from the atmosphere contaminated by the gas into the fresh air.

Ammonia may be tried as a respiratory stimulant. If he has ceased to breathe, artificial respiration should be started.

The best treatment is inhalation of oxygen or a mixture of oxygen and carbon dioxide, and removal to hospital should be as prompt as possible.

Treatment for a Person suffering from Electric Shock. If the patient is still in contact with the electrical circuit and the current cannot be cut off, efforts must be made to pull him away from the live wire.

It is necessary to insulate the hands in some way, other-wise the current will pass from the victim to the would-be rescuer. First of all it should be remembered that water is a good conductor of electricity, therefore, if the ground is damp the rescuer should stand on a piece of dry wood, or on a thick woollen coat or rug. The patient should be grasped by the clothing and the rescuer's hands be protected with some insulating dry substance, such as any rubber material, folds of dry newspaper or clothing. If the patient cannot readily be reached, as, for example, if the accident occurred on an electric railway, he might be dragged from the live rail with the aid of wooden walking sticks with crooked handles. Umbrellas are dangerous on account of the metal spokes; all metals are good conductors of electricity.

If these efforts are successful, the first treatment to apply is artificial respiration. The burns sustained by the patient will have to be treated later.

Suggestions for further reading:

The Treatment of Wound Shock, Medical Research Council
    Memorandum No. 34.
British Red Cross Society—Manual of First-Aid.

INDEX

MADE AND PRINTED BY OFF-SET IN GREAT BRITAIN BY
WILLIAM CLOWES AND SONS, LIMITED, LONDON AND BECCLES,
FOR BAILLIÈRE, TINDALL AND COX, LIMITED

REFERENCE BOOKS

• • • • • • • • • • • • • • • • •

BAILLIÈRE'S NURSES' DICTIONARY

Revised by BARBARA F. CAPE, S.R.N., S.C.M., D.N.

A new edition of this ever-popular dictionary, thoroughly revised and brought up-to-date. The 26 appendixes of "Essential Information" are a special feature.

Fifteenth Edition. 550 pages, 507 drawings.

7s. 6d. *Postage and packing 9d.*

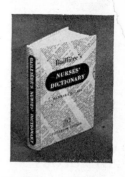

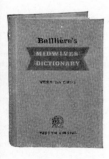

BAILLIÈRE'S MIDWIVES' DICTIONARY

VERA DA CRUZ, S.R.N., S.C.M., M.T.D.

The ideal pocket-sized dictionary for the obstetric nurse. "A little mine of invaluable information . . . it really does contain the exact definition wanted in a hurry."— *The Midwives' Chronicle.*

Fourth Edition. 415 pages, 145 illustrations.

An appendix of essential information in 35 sections.

7s. 6d. *Postage and packing 9d.*

BAILLIÈRE'S POCKET BOOK OF WARD INFORMATION

Revised by MARJORIE HOUGHTON, O.B.E., S.R.N., S.C.M., D.N.

Contents include:
Weights and Measures, Dosage and Solution Strengths, Thermometers, Pharmaceutical Preparations, Classification of Drugs, Prescription Abbreviations, Dangerous Drugs, Dosages, Antibiotics, Hormones, Treatment of Poisoning, Sterilization, Disinfectants and Antiseptics, Enemas, X-rays, Maintaining Respiration, Oxygen Therapy, Fluid Balance, Blood Transfusion, Urine Testing, Laboratory Tests, Calories.

Tenth Edition. 216 pages.

6s. 6d. *Postage and packing 9d.*

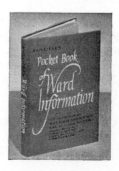

Nurses' Aids Series

A series of complete illustrated textbooks covering the requirements of the G.N.C. Examination syllabus, each volume being written by an expert on the subject. New volumes or editions may have been added; up-to-date information will gladly be supplied on request.

Aids to:

ANATOMY AND PHYSIOLOGY

By Katharine F. Armstrong, S.R.N., S.C.M., D.N., formerly Sister Tutor, King's College Hospital, London.
6th Ed. 9s. 6d.

HYGIENE FOR NURSES

By Edith M. Funnell, S.R.N., D.N., formerly Sister Tutor, Royal Sussex County Hpl., Brighton. *5th Ed.* 7s. 6d.

PRACTICAL NURSING

By Marjorie Houghton, O.B.E., S.R.N., S.C.M., D.N., formerly Sister Tutor, University College Hospital, London.
9th Ed. 8s. 6d.

PSYCHOLOGY FOR NURSES

By A. Altschul. B.A., S.R.N., R.M.N., Principal Tutor, Bethlem Royal Hospital, London. 10s. 6d.

ARITHMETIC IN NURSING

By Wm. C. Fream, S.R.N., B.T.A., CERT. Tutor, General Hpl., Lagos.
2nd Ed. 7s. 6d.

TRAY AND TROLLEY SETTING

By Marjorie Houghton, O.B.E., S.R.N. S.C.M., D.N., formerly Sister Tutor University College Hospital, London
6th Ed. 8s. 6d

MEDICAL NURSING

By Marjorie Houghton, O.B.E., S.R.N. S.C.M., D.N., formerly Sister Tutor, University College Hospital, London, and Mary Whittow, S.R.N., Ward Sister Medical Unit, University College Hospital, London. *6th Ed.* 12s. 6d

SURGICAL NURSING

By Katharine F. Armstrong, S.R.N., S.C.M. D.N., formerly Sister Tutor, King's College Hospital. London, and Norma Jamieson, M.A., S.R.N., S.C.M., Sister Tutor. St. Thomas's Hospital, London.
7th Ed. 12s. 6d

OBSTETRIC AND GYNÆCOLOGICAL NURSING

By Hilda M. Gration, S.R.N., S.C.M., D.N. formerly Sister Tutor, Guy's Hospital London, and Dorothy L. Holland, S.R.N. S.C.M., D.N., formerly Sister Tutor, Guy's Hospital, London. *6th Ed.* 8s. 6d

MATERIA MEDICA FOR NURSES

By Amy E. Squibbs, S.R.N., D.N., Sister Tutor, General Infirmary, Leeds
5th Ed. 8s. 6

Baillière's Anato

TO SEE IS TO LEARN! That is why Baillière's Atlases of the Male and Female Anatomy are so valuable for they enable you to see the relative size, shape, position and detail of every part and structure of the human body. Each atlas has a key naming every part and a clear and concise text explaining and

Atlas of Female Anatomy

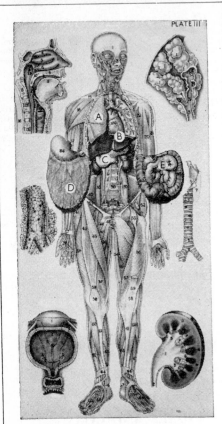

Five plates, printed in full colour.

Note in the illustration of Plate III on the left the letters A, B, C, D and E on certain organs. The organs so lettered are designed to lift up, thus enabling the organs beneath to be seen. By this means the relationship of the internal organs can be learnt *at a glance.* This unique feature makes learning by seeing easy, for not only is each internal organ fully visible, so that its shape and size may be memorised, but its exact position and relationship to other organs is made abundantly clear. The plates printed in full colour teach by seeing, and the text accompanying the plates explains how the parts of the body function. For studying the male anatomy see the description of Baillière's Atlas of the Male Anatomy

Price 12s. 6d. ea

"*The be*

mical Atlases

teaching the anatomy and physiology of the body is also included. Printed in full colour. Size 17 in. × 8½ in. each. By Miss Katharine Armstrong, S.R.N., S.C.M., D.N., and Douglas J. Kidd, M.M.A.A.

Atlas of Male Anatomy

Four coloured and three black and white plates.

To study human anatomy it is essential to consider both the male and the female body. That is why it is necessary to have two Atlases. The Male Atlas is just as important and essential as the Female Atlas. See how clearly (in spite of its reduced size) every detail stands out in the illustration of Plate IV on the right, which is printed in full colour in the atlas and shows the vascular system, the veins and arteries, the heart in various aspects, the pelvic contents etc. Plate IV is another example of "To see is to learn", and studied with the simple, clear explanatory text, learning becomes easy. To all who have to study anatomy Baillière's Atlases of the Male and Female body are indispensable.

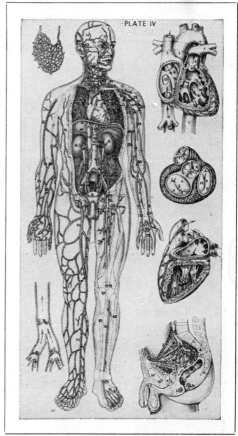

Postage 1s. each

Atlases published"

Handbooks for Nurses . . . .

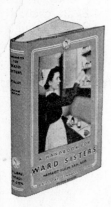

A HANDBOOK FOR WARD SISTERS
MARGARET SCALES, S.R.N., S.C.M.

A book, specially written for this Series, and covering every aspect of ward administration—equipment, personnel, hygiene, nursing routines, reports, and the place of the ward in the hospital as a whole. An essential item of equipment for the table of every Ward Sister.

Second Edition. 328 pages, 43 illus.

21s. *Postage and packing 2s.*

OCCUPATIONAL HEALTH NURSING
F. H. TYRER, M.A., M.R.C.S., L.R.C.P., D.H.

... is a handbook designed to meet the needs of nurses working for the Occupational Health Nursing Certificate of the Royal College of Nursing and the Birmingham Accident Hospital, while nurses already working in industry will find it extremely useful, for in addition to covering medical and nursing fields it also includes such important subjects as Law and Sociology.

184 pages.   Many illustrations.

25s. *Postage and packing 2s.*

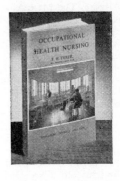

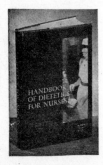

HANDBOOK OF DIETETICS FOR NURSES
CATHERINE F. HARRIS, S.R.N.

A new and enlarged edition of a handbook written to cover the G.N.C. Syllabus, which will give the nurse a full understanding of the therapeutic value and use of food and diets. The principles of dietetic science and their practical application are fully covered, and specimen diet sheets are given for every condition known to benefit from dietetic treatment.

Second Edition. 288 pages. 6 pages of plates.

25s. *Postage and packing 2s.*

DISTRICT NURSING

ELEANOR J. MERRY, O.B.E., S.R.N., S.C.M.,
M.C.S.P., Q.N. & H.V. CERT., and IRIS D.
IRVEN, S.R.N., S.C.M., Q.N. & H.V. CERT.

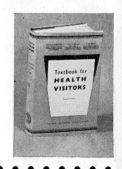

"This book has been well thought out and very well
illustrated, and is a comprehensive study of district
nursing obviously written by those who have had a wide
experience of the practical work. It will be invaluable to
the district nurse for study and should be in the library
of every general hospital."—*Nursing Times*.

Third Edition. **25s.**
Postage 2s.

A HANDBOOK OF CHEST SURGERY FOR NURSES

J. LEIGH COLLIS, M.D., B.Sc., F.R.C.S., and
L. E. MABBIT, S.R.N.

"With the subject matter of this book as her basic knowledge the nurse should find no difficulty in understanding
and carrying out any kind of treatment prescribed by the
surgeon."—*Nursing Times*.

Fourth Edition. 204 pages, 14 plates and 120
other illus.

15s. *Postage and packing* 1s. 6d.

A TEXTBOOK FOR HEALTH VISITORS

LLYWELYN ROBERTS, M.D. (Hygiene),
M.R.C.P., D.P.H., C. H. SHAW, M.D., M.R.C.S.,
D.P.H. and BERYL D. CORNER, M.D., F.R.C.P.

The only book covering the full requirements of the
Health Visitors' Certificate Examination. "An admirable
basic textbook . . . the field covered appears complete."
—*Nursing Mirror*.

Second Edition.
32s. 6d. *Postage and packing* 2s. 6d.

A library of textbooks specially written for the
trained nurse who is studying for specialist
qualifications or appointments and for the
young nurse who is just beginning her training
in a particular field.

All prices are liable to alteration.

Baillière's Handbooks

. . . .

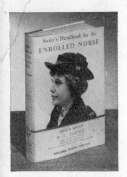

SWIRE'S HANDBOOK FOR THE ENROLLED NURSE

Revised by R. THORA FARNOL, S.R.N., S.C.M., D.N.

The only textbook of its kind written expressly for the assistant nurse with a full appreciation of her needs derived from practical experience. Covers the syllabus of the G.N.C. and provides a basis of practical knowledge for both training and after-years.

Fourth Edition. 348 pages, 185 illustrations.

16s. *Postage and packing* 1s. 6d.

MAYES' HANDBOOK FOR MIDWIVES AND MATERNITY NURSES

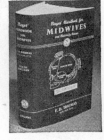

Revised by F. D. THOMAS, S.R.N., S.C.M., M.T.D.

"Packed with sound advice and instruction . . . the author's succinct manner of teaching is admirably demonstrated throughout . . . profusely illustrated. Practising midwives will find this handbook a mine of information."—*Nursing Times.*

Sixth Edition. 478 pages, 19 plates and 167 illus.

22s. 6d. *Postage and packing* 2s.

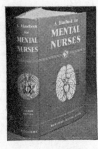

A HANDBOOK FOR MENTAL NURSES

Published in association with The Royal Medico-Psychological Association.

The only complete handbook dealing with the subject, and covering every aspect of mental nursing. A full description is given of modern techniques and method of treatment with a clear explanation of the nurse/patient relationship.

There is an index and glossary of unusual technical terms.

Eighth Edition. 496 pages, 26 illus. (4 in colour).

21s. *Postage and packing* 2s.

BERKELEY'S PICTORIAL MIDWIFERY

Revised by D. M. STERN, M.A., M.B., Ch.B., F.R.C.S., F.R.C.O.G.

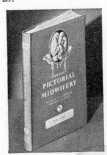

A pictorial survey with excellent illustrations accompanied by clear descriptive text, which will prove invaluable to the pupil midwife, and to the qualified midwife. Really a *must* for any midwife.

Fifth Edition. 176 pages, with 2 coloured plates and 224 drawings.

15s. *Postage and packing* 1s. 6d.